CANCER PROGNOSIS

Edited by **Guy-Joseph Lemamy**

Cancer Prognosis
http://dx.doi.org/10.5772/intechopen.73142
Edited by Guy-Joseph Lemamy

Contributors

Pandurangan Ramaraj, Xi-Dai Long, Daniela Furrer, Caroline Diorio, Claudie Paquet, Simon Jacob, Guy-Joseph Lemamy

Notice

Statements and opinions expressed in the chapters are these of the individual contributors and not necessarily those of the editors or publisher. No responsibility is accepted for the accuracy of information contained in the published chapters. The publisher assumes no responsibility for any damage or injury to persons or property arising out of the use of any materials, instructions, methods or ideas contained in the book.

First published in London, United Kingdom, 2018 by IntechOpen
IntechOpen is the global imprint of INTECHOPEN LIMITED, registered in England and Wales, registration number: 11086078, The Shard, 25th floor, 32 London Bridge Street
London, SE19SG – United Kingdom
Printed in Croatia

British Library Cataloguing-in-Publication Data
A catalogue record for this book is available from the British Library

Additional hard copies can be obtained from orders@intechopen.com

Cancer Prognosis, Edited by Guy-Joseph Lemamy
p. cm.
Print ISBN 978-1-78984-774-1
Online ISBN 978-1-78984-775-8

We are IntechOpen,
the world's leading publisher of
Open Access books
Built by scientists, for scientists

3,900+
Open access books available

116,000+
International authors and editors

120M+
Downloads

Our authors are among the

151
Countries delivered to

Top 1%
most cited scientists

12.2%
Contributors from top 500 universities

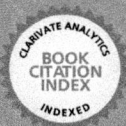

Interested in publishing with us?
Contact book.department@intechopen.com

Numbers displayed above are based on latest data collected.
For more information visit www.intechopen.com

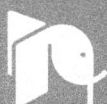

Meet the editor

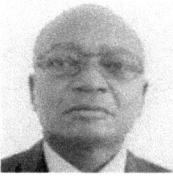

Guy-Joseph Lemamy, PhD, is currently a professor in the Department of Cellular and Molecular Biology-Genetics, and Director of the Laboratory of Cellular and Molecular Biopathologies, at the Faculty of Medicine, Université des Sciences de la Santé (USS), Libreville, Gabon. Dr. Lemamy obtained his PhD in Biochemistry and Cell Biology at the Faculty of Medicine, Université Montpellier 1, France. His PhD thesis work concerned the search for new tumor markers in breast cancers, led by the Medical Research Institute (INSERM U148) in Montpellier, France. Dr. Lemamy is the author of many book chapters and journal articles about tumor markers and is involved in other scientific activities, such as membership of the Scientific Advisory Board of Gabon Scientific Research Guiding Plan.

Contents

Introduction

Introductory Chapter: Genes Expression in the Control of Cell Cycle and Their Potential Value in Cancer Prognosis

Guy Joseph Lemamy

Additional information is available at the end of the chapter

http://dx.doi.org/10.5772/intechopen.81917

1. Introduction

The human body is made of up to trillions of cells. Those cells respond to three characteristics: the differentiation into up to 200 different cellular types which acquire specific functions, the cooperation between those cells using various signaling pathways to sustain the body's physiological unity, and the genetic programming of cell death (the apoptosis). The programmed cell death goes hand in hand with the sustainability of life highlighted at the cell level by the "immortality" of cancer cells, the permanent renewal process of certain tissues such as those of the intestine and blood, as well as the sustainability of the species.

The cancer is a genomic disease in which the early stage is represented by activation of oncogene and inactivation of suppressor genes, which result in transformed cells that grow out of cell cycle control. Two families of genes, the oncogenes and antioncogenes (also called tumor suppressor genes), cause and accelerate the carcinogenesis process when their structure or the regulation of their expression is altered. These genes are equivalent in cancer etiology but differ themselves by their functions and by the mechanisms of their activation. The expression of oncogenes and antioncogenes, respectively, controls in a positive and negative way the cell cycle progression [1] (**Figure 1**).

Among the oncogenes, HER2 is involved in the early stages of carcinogenesis. HER2 is located on chromosome 17 [2] and codes for a transmembrane tyrosine kinase receptor that belongs to a family of four members: human epidermal growth factor receptor (HER) [3]. HER is activated after the binding of its ligand which allows the phosphorylation of tyrosine residues in the intracellular domain of the receptor. This activation leads to signaling pathways promoting cell proliferation, survival, migration, adhesion, angiogenesis, or differentiation

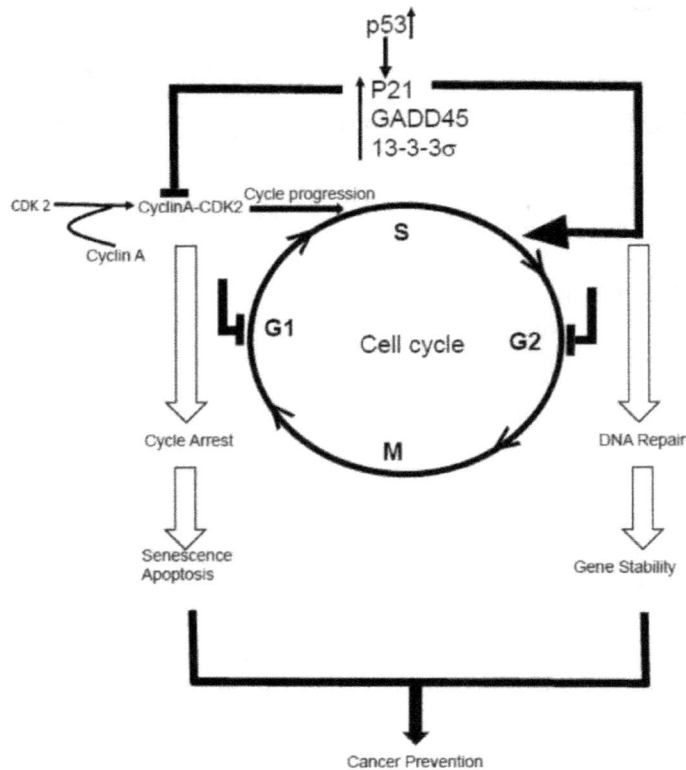

Figure 1. Signaling pathways of p53 in gene stability and cancer prevention. DNA damage increases p53 protein levels that stimulate expression of various genes such as p21, GADD45, or 13-3-3σ. The progression of cell cycle activated by cyclin-CDK complexes is temporarily inhibited by the resulting proteins at the G1 and G2 phases (⊣). Meanwhile, the exonuclease activity of p53 helps to repair damaged DNA. Cells with serious DNA mutations are directed to senescence or apoptosis.

[4]. In breast cancer cells, HER2 gene is amplified followed by the protein overexpression [5]. HER2 overexpression enhances cell proliferation through rapid degradation of the cyclin-dependent kinase (CdK) inhibitor p27 and the upregulation of factors that promote cell cycle progression such as CdK6 and cyclins D1 and E. HER2 is used as prognostic, prognosis, and predictive biomarker in breast cancer [6] (**Figure 2**).

In human cancer, the p53 tumor suppressor gene is the most commonly mutated gene. The p53 gene is mapped to the region 17p13.1, on the short arm of chromosome 17 [7], and codes for the p53 protein (tumor protein of 53 kDa) [8]. The p53 protein plays a main role in cell cycle control and cancer prevention. Damages in DNA occurring during the cell cycle or oncogene activation induce the p53 protein accumulation, resulting in temporary cell cycle arrest at the G1 and G2 checkpoints, DNA repair, differentiation, senescence, apoptosis, or antiangiogenesis. The p53 protein stimulates the expression of other genes such as p21, growth arrest and DNA damage-inducible 45 proteins (GADD45), 13-3-3σ, etc. These proteins are implicated in inactivation of cyclin-cyclin-dependent kinase (cyclin-CDK) complexes required for the progression of the cell cycle (**Figure 1**).

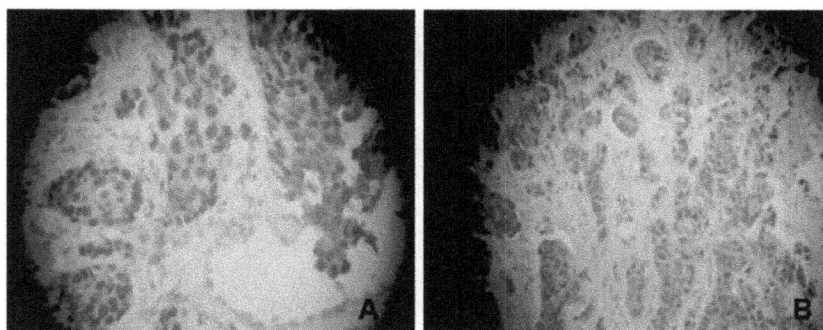

Figure 2. Immunostaining (brown) of estrogen receptor (ER) and HER2 in ductal invasive breast carcinoma. ER (A) and HER2 (B) were revealed, respectively, by their specific antibody. The tissue was counterstained by hematoxylin (blue). Magnification by light microscopy ×400 (from collaboration between Department of Surgical Pathology and Department of Cellular and Molecular Biology-Genetics; Faculty of Medicine, University of Health Sciences, Libreville, Gabon).

In breast cancer, other tumor suppressor genes such as BRCA1 or BRCA2 [9–11] code for proteins that repair DNA damages. Mutations of these genes result in mutated proteins that cannot repair DNA, and cells bearing such mutations will turn into cancers. Taken together, the mutations of BRCA1 and BRCA2 cause about 20–25% of inherited breast cancer and 5–10% of all cancers [12].

Breast cancer risk is of about 50–80% in women with a genetic predisposition [13, 14]. Furthermore, it has been shown that mutation of BRCA1 and BRCA2 is a predictive factor of a major risk of breast cancer [15].The tumor progression can be locally favored by mitogenic effects of hormones, or growth factors which stimulate the tumor's growth, or by activating vascular endothelial growth factor (VEGF) receptor to induce angiogenesis. Human breast cancer is characterized by its high sensitivity to estrogens and its high metastatic potential. About 50% of these cancers are sensitive to antiestrogen treatment [16]. Therefore, the presence of estrogen receptor (ER) is considered to be a predictive factor of response to hormone therapy. Moreover, ER has been shown to be an independent prognostic factor in mammary cancer [16] (**Figure 2**).

Furthermore, estrogens and growth factors induce proteases such as cathepsin D [17]. Cathepsin D is an acid aspartyl endoprotease that is routed through the trans-Golgi network (TGN), by binding to the mannose-6-phosphate/insulin-like growth factor 2 receptor (M6P/IGF2-R) via M6P signals, to lysosomes for degradation. In cancer cells, cathepsin D acts as mitogen promoting metastases [18, 19] and tumor angiogenesis [20, 21]. Clinical studies revealed that cathepsin D is an independent prognostic factor for metastasis risk in breast cancer [22]. In parallel, experimental studies in breast cancer cell lines showed deficiencies of cathepsin D routing to lysosomes, suggesting defects at the receptor level.

Therefore, the M6P/IGF2-R has been hypothesized as being coded by a breast cancer suppressor gene [23], and its potential prognostic significance in breast cancer has been suggested [24].

The cancer pathology includes more than 100 diseases that can cause serious illness or death if not detected in time. The purpose of this book is to present current developments in the methodology in cell and molecular biology which have deeply advanced in the understanding of cancer's prevention and prognosis. Among them, the research for biomarkers may be essential since they can be the target of a preventive therapy, a marker of risk that can be used to identify populations with high risk or a marker of a drug's toxicity used in prevention which can help to monitor its tolerance.

Author details

Guy Joseph Lemamy

Address all correspondence to: guylemamy@yahoo.fr

Department of Cellular and Molecular Biology – Genetics, Faculty of Medicine, University of Health Sciences (Université des Sciences de la Santé - USS), Libreville, Gabon

References

[1] Weinberg RA. Positive and negative control on cell growth. Biochemistry. 1989;**28**: 8263-8269

[2] Popescu NC, King CR, Kraus MH. Localization of the human erbB-2 gene on normal and rearranged chromosomes 17 to bands q12-21.32. Genomics. 1898;**4**(3):362-366

[3] Yarden Y, Sliwkowski MX. Untangling the erbB-2 gene signaling network. Nature Reviews. Molecular Cell Biology. 2001;**2**(2):127-137

[4] Moasser MM. The oncogene HER2: Its signaling and transforming functions and its role in human cancer pathogenesis. Oncogene. 2007;**26**(45):6469-6487

[5] Kallioniemi OP, Kallioniemi A, Kurisu W, Thor A, Chen LC, Smith HS, et al. ERBB2 amplification in breast cancer analyzed by fluorescence in situ hybridization. Proceedings of the National Academy of Sciences of the United States of America. 1992;**89**(12): 5321-5325

[6] Esteva FJ, Yu D, Hung MC, Hortobagyi GN. Molecular predictors of response to trastuzumab and lapatinib in breast cancer. Nature Reviews. Clinical Oncology. 2010;**7**(2): 98-107

[7] Benchimol S, Lamb P, Crawford LV, Sheer D, Shows TB, Bruns GA, et al. Transformation associated p53 protein os encoded by a gene on human chromosome 17. Somatic Cell and Molecular Genetics. 1985;**11**:505-510

[8] Lane DP, Crawford LV. T antigen is bound to a host protein in SV40 transformed cells. Nature. 1979;**278**:261-263

[9] Hall JM, Lee MK, Newman B, Morrow JE, Anderson LA, Huey B, et al. Linkage of early-onset familial breast cancer to chromosome 17q21. Science. 1990;**250**:1684-1689

[10]   Miki Y, Swensen J, Shattuck-Eidens D, Futreal PA, Harshman K, Tavtigian S, et al. A strong candidate for the breast and ovarian cancer susceptibility gene BRCA1. Science. 1994;**266**:66-71

[11]   Wooster R, Neuhausen SL, Mangion J, Quirk Y, Ford D, Collins N, et al. Localization of a breast cancer susceptibility gene, BRCA2 to chromosome 13q12-13. Science. 1994;**265**:2088-2090

[12]   Easton DF, Bishop DT, Ford D, Crockford GP. Breast cancer linkage consortium. Genetic linkage analysis in familial breast and ovarian cancer: Results from 214 families. American Journal of Human Genetics. 1993;**52**:678-701

[13]   Antoniou A, Pharoah PD, Narod S, et al. Average risks of breast and ovarian cancer associated with BRCA1 or BRCA2 mutations detected in case series unselected for family history: A combined analysis of 22 studies. American Journal of Human Genetics. 2003;**72**:1117-1130

[14]   Ford D, Easton DF, Stratton M, et al. Genetic heterogeneity and penetrance analysis of the BRCA1 and BRCA2 genes in breast cancer families. The breast cancer consortium. American Journal of Human Genetics. 1998;**62**:676-689

[15]   Eiseinger F, Bressac B, Castaigne D, et al. Identification and management of hereditary predisposition to cancer of the breast and ovary (update 2004). Bulletin du Cancer. 2004;**91**(3):219-237

[16]   McGuire WL. Hormone receptor: Their role in predicting prognosis and response to endocrine therapy. Seminars in Oncology. 1978;**5**:2428-2433

[17]   Cavaillès V, Augereau P, Garcia M, Rochefort H. Estrogens and growth factors induce the mRNA of the 52K-pro-Cathepsin D secreted by breast cancer cells. Nucleic Acids Research. 1988;**16**:1903-1919

[18]   Garcia M, Derocq D, Pujol P, Rochefort H. Overexpression of transfected Cathepsin D in transformed cells increases their malignant phenotype and metastatic potency. Oncogene. 1990;**5**(12):1809-1814

[19]   Vetvicka V, Vetvickova J, Fusek M. Effect of human procathepsin D on proliferation of human cell lines. Cancer Letters. 1994;**79**(2):131-135

[20]   Berchem G, Glondu M, Gleize M, Brouillet JP, Vignon F, Garcia M, et al. Cathepsin D affects multiple tumor progression steps in vivo: Proliferation, angiogenesis and apoptosis. Oncogene. 2002;**21**(38):5951-5055

[21]   Laurent-Matha V, Maruani-Herman S, Prébois C, Beaujoin M, Glondu M, Noël A, et al. Catalytically inactive human Cathepsin D triggers fibroblast invasive growth. The Journal of Cell Biology. 2005;**168**(3):489-499

[22]   Spyratos F, Maudelone T, Brouillet JP, Brunet M, Andrieu C, Defrenne A, et al. Cathepsin D: An independent prognostic factor for metastasis of breast cancer. The Lancet. 1989;ii:1115-1118

[23] Lemamy GJ, Esslimani S, Berthe ML, Roger P. Is the Mannose-6-phosphate/insulin-like growth factor 2 receptor (M6P/IGF2-R) coded by a breast cancer suppressor gene? Advances in Experimental Medicine and Biology. 2008;**617**:305-310

[24] Lemamy GJ, Roger P, Mani JC, Robert M, Rochefort H, Brouillet JP. High-affinity anti-bodies from hen's-egg yolks against human mannose-6-phosphate/insulin-like growth factor 2 receptor (M6P/IGF2-R): Characterization and potential use in clinical cancer studies. International Journal of Cancer. 1999;**80**:896-902

Molecular Markers Studies

The Human Epidermal Growth Factor Receptor 2 (HER2) as a Prognostic and Predictive Biomarker: Molecular Insights into HER2 Activation and Diagnostic Implications

Daniela Furrer, Claudie Paquet, Simon Jacob and Caroline Diorio

Additional information is available at the end of the chapter

http://dx.doi.org/10.5772/intechopen.78271

Abstract

The human epidermal growth factor receptor 2 (HER2) is a transmembrane tyrosine kinase receptor protein. *HER2* gene amplification and receptor overexpression, which occur in 15–20% of breast cancer patients, are important markers for poor prognosis. Moreover, HER2-positive status is considered a predictive marker of response to HER2 inhibitors including trastuzumab and lapatinib. Therefore, reliable HER2 determination is essential to determine the eligibility of breast cancer patients to targeted anti-HER2 therapies. In this chapter, we aim to illustrate important aspects of the HER2 receptor as well as the molecular consequences of its aberrant constitutive activation in breast cancer. In addition, we will present the methods that can be used for the evaluation of HER2 status at different levels (protein, RNA, and DNA level) in clinical practice.

Keywords: breast neoplasm, oncogene, tyrosine kinase receptor, molecular oncology, HER2 status, HER2 inhibitors

1. Introduction

Breast cancer is the most frequently diagnosed cancer among women worldwide, affecting over 1.5 million women each year. In 2015, it is estimated that worldwide 500,000 women have died from this malignancy, which represents 15% of all cancer-related deaths among women [1].

It is now well recognized that breast cancer comprises a heterogeneous group of diseases in term of differentiation and proliferation, prognosis and treatment. Over the past decades, microarray-based gene expression studies have allowed the identification of breast cancer intrinsic subtypes [2–4]. One of these subtypes is the so-called human epidermal growth factor receptor 2 (HER2)-enriched subtype. HER2 is a transmembrane tyrosine kinase receptor [5]. This protein is encoded by the *HER2* gene, which is located on the long arm of chromosome 17 (17q12–21.32) [6]. The HER2-enriched subtype is characterized by high expression of HER2 and other genes of the 17q amplicon, including growth factor receptor bound protein 7 (GRB7), and low to intermediate expression of luminal genes such as Estrogen Receptor 1 (ESR1) and Progesterone Receptor (PGR) [7]. Clinically, HER2-positive breast cancer occurs in 15–20% of breast cancer patients and is characterized by the overexpression of the HER2 receptor and/or *HER2* gene amplification [8]. HER2-positive breast cancer patients have a particular worse prognosis. Importantly, HER2-positive breast cancer patients are eligible to receive targeted treatment with trastuzumab, a monoclonal antibody specifically directed against the HER2 receptor [9]. Trastuzumab treatment, in combination with chemotherapy, improves the outcome of early [10, 11] and metastatic [12, 13] HER2-positive breast cancer patients. The US Food and Drug Administration (FDA) approved trastuzumab for the treatment of metastatic HER2-positive breast cancer patients in 1998 and for the treatment of early HER2-positive breast cancer patients in 2006. Lapatinib is a small-molecule inhibitor of the intracellular tyrosine kinase domain of both HER2 and EGFR receptors [14]. Lapatinib has received FDA approval in 2007 as combination therapy with capecitabine for the treatment of patients with HER2-positive advanced breast cancer patients who had progressed on trastuzumab-based regimens [15]. Although anti-HER2 agents are generally well tolerated, trastuzumab administration has been associated with cardiac side effects, especially when used in combination with anthracyclines [16].

HER2 plays a significant role in breast cancer pathogenesis. It is therefore essential to understand the biology of this receptor in order to better treat HER2-positive breast cancer patients. Evaluation of HER2 status in breast cancer specimens raises several technical considerations. In the last decades, several methods have been developed for HER2 assessment. In this article, we will review important aspects of the HER2 biology and its relevance in breast cancer and present the techniques that are used in clinical practice for the determination of HER2 status in breast cancer specimens.

2. HER2 biology and methods of assessment of HER2 status

2.1. HER2 receptor

The HER2 receptor is a 185 kDa transmembrane protein that is encoded by the *HER2* (also known as *erb-b2 receptor tyrosine kinase 2 [ERBB2]*) gene, which is located on the long arm of chromosome 17 (17q12–21.32) [6]. HER2 is normally expressed on cell membranes of epithelial cells of several organs like the breast and the skin, as well as gastrointestinal, respiratory, reproductive, and urinary tract [17]. In normal breast epithelial cells, HER2 is expressed at low levels (two copies of the *HER2* gene and up to 20,000 HER2 receptors) [18], whereas in HER2-positive breast cancer cells, there is an increase in the number of *HER2* gene copies (up to 25–50, termed gene amplification) and HER2 receptors (up to 40 to 100 fold increase, termed protein overexpression), resulting in up to 2 million receptors expressed at the tumor cell surface [19]. Besides breast cancer, HER2 overexpression has also been reported in other types of tumors, including stomach, ovary, colon, bladder, lung, uterine cervix, head and neck, and esophageal cancer as well as uterine serous endometrial carcinoma [20].

2.1.1. HER2 structure and function

HER2 belongs to the epidermal growth factor receptor (EGFR) family. This family is composed of four HER receptors: human epidermal growth factor receptor 1 (HER1) (also termed EGFR), HER2, human epidermal growth factor receptor 3 (HER3), and human epidermal growth factor receptor 4 (HER4) [5].

HER family members are transmembrane receptor tyrosine kinases. Tyrosine kinases are enzymes that carry out tyrosine phosphorylation, namely the transfer of the γ phosphate of adenosine triphosphate (ATP) to tyrosine residues on protein substrate [21].

HER receptors share a similar structure. They are composed of an extracellular domain (ECD), a transmembrane segment and an intracellular region [22]. The ECD domain is divided into four parts: domains I and III, which play a role in ligand binding, and domains II and IV, which contain several cysteine residues that are important for disulfide bond formation [23]. The transmembrane segment is composed of 19–25 amino acid residues. The intracellular region is composed of a juxtamembrane segment, a functional protein kinase domain (with the exception of HER3 that lacks tyrosine kinase activity [24] and must partner with another family member to be activated [25]), and a C-terminal tail containing multiple phosphorylation sites required for propagation of downstream signaling [23]. The catalytic domain contains the ATP binding pocket, a conserved site essential to ATP binding [26].

HER receptors are activated by both homo- and heterodimerization, generally induced by ligand binding [27]. This suggests that HER receptor family has evolved to provide a high degree of signal diversity [28]. The cellular outcome produced by HER receptors activation depends on the signaling pathways that are induced, as well as their magnitude and duration, which are influenced by the composition of the dimer and the identity of the ligand [28].

Several growth factor ligands interact with the HER receptors [29]. HER1 receptor is activated by six ligands: epidermal growth factor (EGF), epigen (EPG), transforming growth factor α (TGFα), amphiregulin, heparin-binding EGF-like growth factor, betacellulin and epiregulin. HER3 and HER4 receptors bind neuregulins (neuregulin-1, neuregulin-2, neuregulin-3, and neuregulin-4). HER2 is a co-receptor for many ligands and is often transactivated by EGF-like ligands, inducing the formation of HER1-HER2 heterodimers. Neuregulins induces the formation of HER2-HER3 and HER2-HER4 heterodimers [29]. However, no known ligand can promote HER2 homodimer formation, implying that no ligand can bind directly to HER2 [30].

The structural basis for receptor dimerization has been elucidated in recent years through crystallographic studies [31, 32]. Dimerization is mediated by the dimerization arm, a region of the extracellular region of HER receptors. While in its inactivated state the dimerization arm of EGFR, HER3 and HER4 is hidden, ligand binding induces a receptor conformational change leading to exposure of the dimerization arm [31]. In contrast to the other three HER receptors, the dimerization arm of the HER2 receptor is permanently partially exposed, thus permitting its dimerization even if the HER2 receptor lacks ligand-binding activity [32].

Interaction between the dimerization arms of two HER receptors promotes the formation of a stable receptor dimer in which the kinase regions of both receptors are closed enough to permit transphosphorylation of tyrosine residues, i.e. the transfer of a phosphate group by a protein kinase to a tyrosine residue in a different kinase molecule [33, 34]. The first member of the dimer mediates the phosphorylation of the second, and the second dimer mediates the phosphorylation of the first [23].

The phosphorylation of specific tyrosine residues following HER receptor activation and the subsequent recruitment and activation of downstream signaling proteins leads to activation of downstream signaling pathways promoting cell proliferation, survival, migration, adhesion, angiogenesis and differentiation [35]. The Phosphatidylinositol 3'-kinase (PI3K)-Akt pathway and the Ras/Raf/MEK/ERK pathway (also known as extracellular signal-regulated kinase/mitogen-activated protein kinase (ERK/MAPK) pathway) are the two most important and most extensively studied downstream signaling pathways that are activated by the HER receptors [5, 36]. These downstream signaling cascades control cell cycle, cell growth and survival, apoptosis, metabolism and angiogenesis [37, 38]. Signaling from HER receptors is then terminated through the internalization of the activated receptors from the cell surface by endocytosis. Internalized receptors are then either recycled back to the plasma membrane (HER2, HER3, HER4) or degraded in lysosomes (HER1) [39, 40].

HER heterodimers produce more potent signal transduction than homodimers. This can be explained by the fact that heterodimerization provides additional phosphotyrosine residues necessary for the recruitment of effector proteins [28]. Heterodimerization follows a strict hierarchical principle with HER2 representing the preferred dimerization and signaling partner for all other members of the HER family [41]. HER2 seems to function mainly as a co-receptor, increasing the affinity of ligand binding to dimerized receptor complexes [42, 43]. HER2 has the strongest catalytic kinase activity [41] and HER2-containing heterodimers produce intracellular signals that are significantly stronger than signals generated from other HER heterodimers [44]. The HER2-HER3 heterodimer in particular exhibits extremely potent mitogenic activity through the stimulation of the PI3K/Akt pathway, a master regulator of cell growth and survival [45]. Furthermore, HER2 containing heterodimers have a slow rate of receptor internalization, which results in prolonged stimulation of downstream signaling pathways [28]. HER2 can also be activated by complexing with other membrane receptors, such as Insulin-like growth factor I receptor (IGF-1R) [46].

2.1.2. Consequences of constitutive HER2 receptor activation

Whereas in normal cells the activity of tyrosine kinases is a tightly controlled mechanism, in cancer cells, alterations in tyrosine kinases—overexpression of receptor tyrosine kinase proteins, amplification or mutation in the corresponding gene, abnormal stimulation by autocrine growth factors loop or delayed degradation of activated receptor tyrosine kinase—lead to constitutive kinase activation and therefore to aberrant cellular growth and proliferation [34, 47]. Constitutive activation of HER1, HER2, HER3, IGF-1R, Fibroblast growth factor receptor (FGFR), c-Met, Insulin Receptor (IR), Vascular Endothelial Growth Factor Receptor (VEGFR), Jak kinases and Src have been associated with human cancer [34, 48–52].

Several ways of aberrant activation of HER receptors have been described, including ligand binding, molecular structural alterations, lack of the phosphatase activity, or overexpression of the HER receptor [53].

In HER2-positive tumors, receptor overexpression has been identified as the mechanism of HER2 activation. The increased amount of cell surface HER2 receptors associated with HER2 overexpression leads to increased receptor-receptor interactions, provoking a sustained tyrosine phosphorylation of the kinase domain and therefore constant activation of the signaling pathways. HER2 overexpression also enhances HER2 heterodimerization with HER1 and HER3 [54] resulting in an increased activation of the downstream signaling pathways. It has also been shown that HER2 overexpression leads to enhanced HER1 membrane expression and HER1 signaling activity through interference with the endocytic regulation of HER1 [54–56]. While HER1 undergoes endocytic degradation after ligand-mediated activation and homodimerization, HER1-HER2 heterodimers evade endocytic degradation in favor of the recycling pathway [57, 58], resulting in increased HER1 membrane expression and activity [55, 56, 59].

It has also been reported that HER2 overexpression enhances cell proliferation through the rapid degradation of the cyclin-dependent kinase (Cdk) inhibitor p27 and the upregulation of factors that promote cell cycle progression, including Cdk6 and cyclins D1 and E [60].

Several methods have been developed for the assessment of HER2 status in breast cancer specimens, at the protein level, DNA level, and RNA level. Here below, we present some of the existing techniques that are used for the HER2 determination in clinical practice.

2.2. Methods for the evaluation of HER2 status in breast cancer specimens

2.2.1. HER2 status evaluation at the protein level

2.2.1.1. Immunohistochemistry (IHC)

IHC allows the evaluation of the HER2 protein expression in formalin-fixed, paraffin-embedded (FFPE) tissues using specific antibodies directed against the HER2 receptor protein [61]. HER2 receptor is then visualized with the chromogen 3,3'-diaminobenzidine tetrahydrochloride (DAB) resulting in a brownish membranous staining. Several commercially available diagnostic tests for the determination of HER2 expression have been approved by the FDA: the HercepTest™ kit (DAKO, Glostrup, Denmark), the InSite™ HER2/neu kit (clone CB11; BioGenex Laboratories, San Ramon, CA), the Pathway™ kit (clone 4B5; Ventana Medical Systems, Tucson, AZ), and the Bond Oracle HER2 IHC System (Leica Biosystems, Newcastle, UK).

By this method, it is possible to estimate the number of cells showing membranous staining in the tissue section as well as the intensity of the staining [62]. Membranous staining in the invasive component of specimen is scored on a semi-quantitative scale. According to the American Society of Clinical oncology (ASCO) and the College of American Pathologists (CAP) recommendations for HER2 testing in breast cancer published in 2013, HER2 expression is scored as 0 (no staining or weak/incomplete membrane staining in ≤10% of tumor cells), 1+ (weak, incomplete membrane staining in >10% of tumor cells), 2+ (strong, complete membrane staining in ≤10% of tumor cells or weak/moderate and/or incomplete membrane staining in >10% of tumors cells) or 3+ (strong, complete, homogeneous membrane staining in >10% of tumor cells) [61]. In clinical practice, HER2 immunohistochemical status is evaluated as negative if the immunohistochemical score is 0 or 1+, equivocal is the score is 2+, and positive if the score is 3+. Patients with a positive HER2 status at the IHC are eligible for targeted therapy with HER2 inhibitors. The IHC 2+ category is considered borderline and confirmatory testing using an alternative assay (fluorescence *in situ* hybridization (FISH) or other *in situ* hybridization (ISH) methods, see Section 2.2.2) is required for final determination.

IHC is an easy and relatively inexpensive method [63]. However, this technique can be affected by numerous factors, including warm/cold ischemic time [64], delay and duration of fixation [65], and antibody used [66, 67]. Moreover, since the interpretation of results is based on semiquantitative scoring, this technique is prone to interobserver variability and therefore to substantial discrepancies in the IHC results, particularly for cases scoring 2+ [68].

2.2.1.2. Enzyme-linked immunosorbent assay (ELISA)

As mentioned before, HER2 receptor is composed of an extracellular domain (ECD), a transmembrane domain, and an intracellular domain with tyrosine kinase activity. The HER2 ECD can be cleaved from the HER2 full-length receptor through matrix metalloproteases and released into the serum [69]. HER2 ECD levels present in serum can be measured using an enzyme-linked immunosorbent assay (ELISA). HER2 ECD is detected using two antibodies that recognize two specific epitopes of the antigen. Several commercially available ELISA assays received FDA approval: the automated ELISA assay Immuno-1 (Siemens Healthcare Diagnostics, Tarrytown, NY), the manual ELISA assay (Siemens Healthcare Diagnostics) in 2000, and the automated ELISA assay ADVIA Centaur (Siemens Healthcare Diagnostics) in 2003 [70].

Although some studies suggest that HER2 ECD levels measured in patient's serum could be used as a biomarker for the monitoring of the disease course and the response of the patient to therapy, the clinical use of the ELISA assay for the evaluation of the HER2 ECD has not yet been widely implemented [71, 72]. This is mainly due to the fact that studies that analyzed the association between HER2 ECD levels and prognostic and predictive factors in breast cancer patients reported conflicting results, depending on which cutoff value was considered or which assay was used [71].

ELISA is an easy and fast method. In addition, given that HER2 ECD can be measured directly in serum, ELISA can be used to monitor the dynamic changes of HER2 status following treatment or over the course of the disease progression [71]. Results obtained by ELISA, however, might not be reliable if the serum samples are from patients under treatment, as trastuzumab present in the patient's serum might compete with the two antibodies used in the assay.

2.2.2. HER2 status evaluation at the DNA level

2.2.2.1. Fluorescence in situ hybridization (FISH)

The FISH technique is a cytogenetic technique that uses fluorescent probes to target specific DNA sequences in FFPE tissue samples [73]. FISH is effectuated either as a single-color assay (*HER2* probe only) to evaluate *HER2* gene copies per nucleus or as a dual-color assay using differentially labeled HER2 and chromosome 17 centromere (chromosome enumeration probe 17, CEP17) probes simultaneously. The dual-color assay allows the determination of the HER2/CEP17 ratio [74]. The HER2/CEP17 ratio is often regarded as a better reflection of the *HER2* amplification status, as the latter may be influenced by abnormal chromosome 17 copy number (mainly polysomy) [75].

The *HER2* gene locus on chromosome 17 is recognized by the HER2 probe, which is labeled with a fluorophore (orange as example). The α satellite DNA sequence located at the centromeric region of chromosome 17 is recognized by a fluorophore-labeled chromosome 17 centromere probe (green as example). Nuclei are then counterstained with 4,6'-diamino-2-phenylindole (DAPI). Fluorescent hybridization signals can be visualized using a fluorescence microscope equipped with appropriate filters (for example Spectrum Orange for locus-specific probe HER2, Spectrum Green for centromeric probe 17, and the UV filter for the DAPI nuclear counterstain) [76].

Three FISH assay kits have been approved by the FDA for the determination of the *HER2* gene amplification in breast cancer specimens: the single-probe INFORM HER2 FISH DNA kit (Ventana Medical Systems), the dual-probe PathVysion HER-2 DNA probe kit (Abbott Molecular, Des Plaines, IL), and the dual-probe HER2 FISH PharmDx kit (DAKO).

According to the 2013 ASCO/CAP guidelines, a case is evaluated as amplified when the mean *HER2* gene copy number is ≥6 signals/nucleus or HER2/CEP17 ratio is ≥2.0, else as equivocal if mean *HER2* gene copy number is ≥4 and <6 signals/nucleus, and else as non-amplified when the mean *HER2* gene copy number is <4 signals/nucleus. In order to adequately evaluate HER2 status, a minimum of 20 tumor cell nuclei are counted in at least two invasive tumor areas. For equivocal FISH specimens, results are confirmed by counting 20 additional cells [61]. Moreover, the equivocal category requires reflex testing with the alternative assay (IHC) on the same specimen for final determination. Reflex testing can also be performed using IHC or ISH methods on an alternative specimen. If specimen is evaluated as equivocal, even after reflex testing, the oncologist may consider targeted treatment.

Although still matter of debate, several researchers consider FISH as being more accurate and reliable than IHC in the assessment of HER2 status in breast cancer specimens [77–80]. In addition, given that DNA is more stable than protein, preanalytical factors have less impact on assay results compared with IHC [81]. Although the FISH technique yields results that are considered more objective and quantitative than immunohistochemical scoring [73, 82], this method is nine times more time-consuming [83] and three times more expensive compared with IHC [84]. In addition, costly equipment is required for signal detection [67]. The FISH assay can be interpreted only by well-trained personnel, as distinguishing invasive breast cancer from breast carcinoma *in situ* under fluorescence is arduous [85].

Moreover, fluorescence signal counting is time consuming. To overcome this limitation, image analysis software for the automated assessment of fluorescence signals has been developed. Several investigators have reported an excellent concordance between HER2/CEP17 ratios calculated through manual counting and those obtained with automated image analysis system [86–88]. Some image analysis systems has been approved by the FDA for the automated determination of *HER2* gene amplification: the Metafer (MetaSystems, Altlussheim, Germany) and the Ariol HER2/neu FISH (Applied Imaging, San Jose, CA). Furthermore, this software allows the storing of captured images [86].

2.2.2.2. Bright-field in situ hybridization (ISH) methods

Given that FISH technology have some limitations, alternative ISH methods have been developed for the assessment of *HER2* gene amplification in breast cancer specimens. Similar to FISH, these methods allow the quantification of *HER2* gene copy number within tumor cell nuclei in FFPE tissues using a DNA probe that specifically recognizes specific DNA sequences. However, whereas the FISH assay is performed with DNA probes that are coupled to a fluorescent detection system, these alternative ISH methods are performed with probes that are coupled to chromogenic (chromogenic ISH [CISH]), or silver detection system (silver-enhanced ISH [ISH]), or a combination of CISH and SISH (bright-field double ISH [BDISH]) [89]. Similar to FISH, ISH methods are performed either as single-color assay or as a dual-color assay.

Since visualization is achieved using other reactions than fluorescence-labeled probe, signals can be evaluated using a standard bright-field microscope, allowing the simultaneous analysis of *HER2* gene amplification and morphologic features of tissues. Moreover, contrary to fluorescent signals that fade over time, bright-field ISH signals are permanent [90]. Here after, we will briefly describe the bright-field ISH methods that are used in clinics.

2.2.2.3. Chromogenic in situ hybridization (CISH)

CISH allows the visualization of target genes in breast cancer tissue sections through peroxidase enzyme-labeled probes [90]. The single-color CISH assay (SPOT-Light HER2 CISH kit; Life Technologies, Carlsbad, CA), and the dual-color CISH assay (HER2 CISH PharmDx kit; Dako) received FDA approval in 2008 and 2011, respectively [61].

With the single-color CISH assay, only the absolute *HER2* gene copy number is evaluated. The hybridized HER2 probe is visualized by DAB as chromogen. *HER2* gene copies are recognizable as brown chromogenic reaction product signals within nuclei. Slides are then counterstained with hematoxylin [82, 91, 92]. HER2 signals are recognizable either as large brownish signal clusters or as numerous individual brownish small signals [92]. Cases with low-level amplification show six to 10 signals per nucleus in more than 50% of breast cancer cells, whereas high-level amplification cases are characterized by a mean *HER2* gene copy number of more than 10 or by large gene copy clusters in more than 50% of breast cancer cell nuclei [92, 93].

The dual-color CISH assay allows the simultaneous visualization of the HER2 and CEP17 probes on the same slide [94]. HER2 probes are visualized using a chromogen (green as example), whereas CEP17 probes are visualized using another chromogen (red as example). Slides are then counterstained with hematoxylin. Results obtained by dual-color CISH are reported as dual-color FISH [61].

The CISH assay is twice cheaper [72] and 1.2 times faster [82] comparatively to FISH. Furthermore, since the CISH assay allows an easier identification of the invasive component compared with FISH, evaluation of CISH signals is less time-consuming than FISH [82, 94]. In addition, tumor heterogeneity is promptly recognizable, even at low magnification [95]. Moreover, the dual-color assay can be performed on an automated slide stainer, improving the reproducibility of the assay [96]. However, the assessment of *HER2* gene copy number can be arduous in tumor regions showing high-level amplification, since overlapping dots lead to formation of signal clusters that are difficult to evaluate [94]. In addition, technical problems, including under- or overfixation, over- or underdigestion of tissue samples can lead to inaccurate results or loss of signals [91, 93].

2.2.2.4. Silver-enhanced in situ hybridization (SISH)

SISH is an automated enzyme metallography assay, in which an enzyme reaction is used to selectively deposit metallic silver from solution at the reaction site to produce a black staining [97]. All steps of the assay are performed on the Ventana BenchMark XT automated slide stainer [98, 99]. HER2 and chromosome 17 analysis is performed on sequential slides [98, 99]. As previously mentioned, HER2 and CEP17 probes are visualized through the process of enzyme metallography. During the process, silver precipitation is deposited in the nucleus, and HER2 or CEP17 signals are visualized as black dots within cell nuclei [99]. Similar to the FISH assay, *HER2* gene amplification status assessed by SISH is reported as a HER2/CEP17 ratio, according to the ASCO/CAP guidelines [61].

Given that the SISH assay is fully automated, this technique is six times faster to perform than the FISH assay [99]. In addition, black SISH signals are easier to evaluate compared with other bright-field ISH techniques [100, 101]. However, to correct for chromosome 17 aneusomy, the hybridization of a further section is required for separate assessment of CEP17 copy number [100].

2.2.2.5. Bright-field double ISH (BDISH)

Bright-field double ISH (BDISH) or dual-color *in situ* hybridization (dual ISH) is a fully automated bright-field ISH assay for the simultaneous determination of HER2 and CEP17 signals on the same FFPE breast cancer tissue sections [100]. This assay combines the visualization of *HER2* gene copies through the deposition of metallic silver particles, similar to the monocolor SISH procedure, with the detection of CEP17 copies with a red chromogen, similar to the CISH assay [102]. HER2 signals are visualized as discrete black spots and the CEP17 signals as red spots in the nuclei. Slides are then counterstained with hematoxylin [100]. *HER2* gene amplification status assessed by BDISH is reported as a HER2/CEP17 ratio, according to the ASCO/CAP guidelines.

This technique is very pertinent especially for cases displaying chromosome 17 aneusomy or intratumoral heterogeneity, as it allows the simultaneous visualization of both HER2 and CEP17 probes on the same slide [100]. Furthermore, as the HER2 signals and CEP17 signals differ in color and size (HER2 black spots are smaller than CEP17 red spots), both signals can be distinguished from each other, even though they colocalize within cell nuclei [100]. Moreover, since this assay is completely automated, results are available within 6 h, in addition of being more reproducible, as risk of human errors are diminished [101]. The BDISH assay presents the same disadvantages as CISH and SISH.

2.2.2.6. Instant-quality FISH (IQFISH) and automated HER2 FISH

Recently, new FISH assays have been developed for the evaluation of *HER2* gene amplification in breast cancer specimens, including instant-quality FISH (IQFISH), which received

FDA approval, and automated *HER2* FISH. In analogy to conventional FISH, these new assays allow the quantitative determination of *HER2* gene amplification. The IQFISH assay is performed in the same way as manual FISH, with the exception of the hybridization buffer (IQFISH buffer), which considerably reduces the time required for the hybridization step (16 times faster) and therefore the total assay time [103, 104]. Moreover, while hybridization buffer provided in conventional FISH assay contain the toxic formamide, the IQFISH buffer is nontoxic [103]. Compared to conventional FISH, automated FISH is less expensive, since the full automation of the assay requires less human intervention [105]. Furthermore, automated FISH enables faster processing of samples and recording [105].

2.2.3. HER2 status evaluation at the RNA level

2.2.3.1. Polymerase chain reaction (PCR)-based assays

Polymerase chain reaction (PCR) is a technique used for the detection of DNA samples through the exponential amplification of target DNA sequences.

Reverse transcription PCR (RT-PCR) assay allows the quantification of mRNA and can be used for the evaluation of HER2 expression in breast cancer specimens in both FFPE and frozen tissues [106, 107]. Extracted mRNA is at first reverse transcribed into complementary DNA (cDNA). cDNA is then measured by quantitative PCR (qPCR). The relative quantitation of *HER2* gene expression is evaluated comparing the target gene expression with that of housekeeping genes. The relative *HER2* gene expression measured in samples is then normalized to a calibrator obtained by mixing RNA from several normal breast tissue specimens. Of note, the Oncotype Dx (Genomic Health, Redwood City, CA) assay is a test based on RT-PCR technology and is used to analyze the expression of 21 genes involved in breast cancer biology, such as *HER2*, ER, and PR. This assay is used to predict the likelihood of breast cancer recurrence in patients with early-stage, node-negative, ER-positive breast cancer [106].

RT-PCR has a large dynamic range, in addition of being a quantitative method. PCR results, however, are often associated with false-negative results due to dilution of amplified tumor cells with surrounding nonamplified stromal cells [108, 109]. In addition, the evaluation of HER2 status at the mRNA level by RT-PCR using FFPE tissues can be problematic, as mRNA integrity can be damaged by several factors, including tissue fixation and storage time [110].

3. Conclusion(s)

HER2 is a prognostic marker in breast cancer. HER2 overexpression and *HER2* gene amplification, which occur in 15–20% of breast cancer patients, cause aberrant constitutive activation of the signaling pathway. This leads to uncontrolled and unregulated cell growth and correlates with poor outcome of HER2-positive breast cancer patients.

In addition, HER2-positive status is considered a predictive marker of response to HER2-targeted drugs, including trastuzumab and lapatinib [111]. Considering the clinical and economic implications of targeted anti-HER2 treatments, reliable HER2 test results are essential.

False negative results would deny the patients access to the potential benefits of trastuzumab, whereas false positive results would expose patients to the potential cardiotoxic side effects of this expensive agent without experiencing any therapeutic advantages [89].

Although several techniques have obtained FDA approval for the HER2 assessment in breast cancer specimens, the ASCO/CAP guidelines recommend performing IHC or ISH methods to determine HER2 status in breast cancer. The optimal method for evaluating HER2 status in breast cancer specimens, however, is still matter of debate, since each method is characterized by its own advantages and disadvantages. Therefore, emphasis must be put on standardization of procedures and quality control assessment of already existing methods. Also, development of new accurate assays should be promoted. Moreover, large clinical trials are needed to identify the technique that most reliably predicts a positive response to HER2 inhibitors.

Acknowledgements

DF received doctoral fellowships from the Fonds de recherche du Québec—Santé (FRQS) and the Laval University Cancer Research. CD is a recipient of the Canadian Breast Cancer Foundation-Canadian Cancer Society Capacity Development award (award #703003) and the FRQS Research Scholar.

Conflict of interest

The authors have no conflicts of interests to declare.

Notes/thanks/other declarations

The authors have no other declarations.

Acronyms and abbreviations

HER2	Human epidermal growth factor receptor 2
GRB7	Growth factor receptor bound protein 7
ESR1	Estrogen Receptor 1
PGR	Progesterone Receptor
FDA	Food and Drug Administration
EGFR	Epidermal growth factor receptor

IHC	Immunohistochemistry
FISH	Fluorescence *in situ* hybridization
ERBB2	erb-b2 receptor tyrosine kinase 2
HER3	Human epidermal growth factor receptor 3
HER4	Human epidermal growth factor receptor 4
ATP	Adenosine triphosphate
ECD	extracellular domain
EGF	Epidermal growth factor
EPG	Epigen
TGFα	Transforming growth factor α
PI3K	Phosphatidylinositol 3'-kinase
ERK	Extracellular signal-regulated kinase
MAPK	Mitogen-activated protein kinase
FGFR	Fibroblast growth factor receptor
IR	Insulin Receptor
VEGFR	Vascular Endothelial Growth Factor Receptor
Cdk	Cyclin-dependent kinase
FFPE	Formalin-fixed, paraffin-embedded
DAB	3,3'-diaminobenzidine tetrahydrochloride
ASCO	American Society of Clinical Oncology
CAP	College of American Pathologists
ELISA	Enzyme-linked immunosorbent assay
CEP17	Chromosome enumeration probe 17
DAPI	4,6'-diamino-2-phenylindole
ISH	*in situ* hybridization
CISH	Chromogenic *in situ* hybridization
SISH	Silver-enhanced *in situ* hybridization
BDISH	Bright-field double ISH
PCR	polymerase chain reaction

RT-PCR	Reverse transcription PCR
cDNA	Complementary DNA
qPCR	Quantitative PCR

Author details

Daniela Furrer[1,2,3], Claudie Paquet[5,6], Simon Jacob[4,5,6] and Caroline Diorio[1,2,3,5]*

*Address all correspondence to: caroline.diorio@crchudequebec.ulaval.ca

1 Cancer Research Center at Laval University, Quebec City, Canada

2 Oncology Axis, CHU of Quebec Research Center, Quebec City, Canada

3 Department of Social and Preventive Medicine, Laval University, Quebec City, Canada

4 Department of Molecular Biology, Medical Biochemistry and Pathology, Laval University, Quebec City, Canada

5 Deschênes-Fabia Center for Breast Diseases, Quebec City, Canada

6 Pathology Service, Saint-Sacrement Hospital, Quebec City, Canada

References

[1] WHO. 2017. Available from: http://www.who.int/cancer/prevention/diagnosis-screening/breast-cancer/en/ [Accessed: 2017-03-23]

[2] Perou CM, Sorlie T, Eisen MB, van de Rijn M, Jeffrey SS, Rees CA, et al. Molecular portraits of human breast tumours. Nature. 2000;**406**(6797):747-752

[3] Sorlie T. Molecular classification of breast tumors: Toward improved diagnostics and treatments. Methods in Molecular Biology. 2007;**360**:91-114

[4] Sorlie T, Tibshirani R, Parker J, Hastie T, Marron JS, Nobel A, et al. Repeated observation of breast tumor subtypes in independent gene expression data sets. Proceedings of the National Academy of Sciences of the United States of America. 2003;**100**(14):8418-8423

[5] Yarden Y, Sliwkowski MX. Untangling the ErbB signalling network. Nature Reviews. Molecular Cell Biology. 2001;**2**(2):127-137

[6] Popescu NC, King CR, Kraus MH. Localization of the human erbB-2 gene on normal and rearranged chromosomes 17 to bands q12-21.32. Genomics. 1989;**4**(3):362-366

[7] Prat A, Pascual T, Adamo B. Intrinsic molecular subtypes of HER2+ breast cancer. Oncotarget. 2017;**8**(43):73362-73363

[8]   Soerjomataram I, Louwman MW, Ribot JG, Roukema JA, Coebergh JW. An overview of prognostic factors for long-term survivors of breast cancer. Breast Cancer Research and Treatment. 2008;**107**(3):309-330

[9]   Yersal O, Barutca S. Biological subtypes of breast cancer: Prognostic and therapeutic implications. World Journal of Clinical Oncology. 2014;**5**(3):412-424

[10] Gianni L, Dafni U, Gelber RD, Azambuja E, Muehlbauer S, Goldhirsch A, et al. Treatment with trastuzumab for 1 year after adjuvant chemotherapy in patients with HER2-positive early breast cancer: A 4-year follow-up of a randomised controlled trial. The Lancet Oncology. 2011;**12**(3):236-244

[11] Piccart-Gebhart MJ, Procter M, Leyland-Jones B, Goldhirsch A, Untch M, Smith I, et al. Trastuzumab after adjuvant chemotherapy in HER2-positive breast cancer. The New England Journal of Medicine. 2005;**353**(16):1659-1672

[12] Seidman AD, Fornier MN, Esteva FJ, Tan L, Kaptain S, Bach A, et al. Weekly trastuzumab and paclitaxel therapy for metastatic breast cancer with analysis of efficacy by HER2 immunophenotype and gene amplification. Journal of Clinical Oncology: Official Journal of the American Society of Clinical Oncology. 2001;**19**(10):2587-2595

[13] Vogel CL, Cobleigh MA, Tripathy D, Gutheil JC, Harris LN, Fehrenbacher L, et al. Efficacy and safety of trastuzumab as a single agent in first-line treatment of HER2-overexpressing metastatic breast cancer. Journal of Clinical Oncology: Official Journal of the American Society of Clinical Oncology. 2002;**20**(3):719-726

[14] Xia W, Mullin RJ, Keith BR, Liu LH, Ma H, Rusnak DW, et al. Anti-tumor activity of GW572016: A dual tyrosine kinase inhibitor blocks EGF activation of EGFR/erbB2 and downstream Erk1/2 and AKT pathways. Oncogene. 2002;**21**(41):6255-6263

[15] Ryan Q, Ibrahim A, Cohen MH, Johnson J, Ko CW, Sridhara R, et al. FDA drug approval summary: Lapatinib in combination with capecitabine for previously treated metastatic breast cancer that overexpresses HER-2. The Oncologist. 2008;**13**(10):1114-1119

[16] Verma S, Ewer MS. Is cardiotoxicity being adequately assessed in current trials of cytotoxic and targeted agents in breast cancer? Annals of Oncology: Official Journal of the European Society for Medical Oncology. 2011;**22**(5):1011-1018

[17] Press MF, Cordon-Cardo C, Slamon DJ. Expression of the HER-2/neu proto-oncogene in normal human adult and fetal tissues. Oncogene. 1990;**5**(7):953-962

[18] Ross JS, Fletcher JA, Bloom KJ, Linette GP, Stec J, Clark E, et al. HER-2/neu testing in breast cancer. American Journal of Clinical Pathology. 2003;**120**(Suppl):S53-S71

[19] Kallioniemi OP, Kallioniemi A, Kurisu W, Thor A, Chen LC, Smith HS, et al. ERBB2 amplification in breast cancer analyzed by fluorescence in situ hybridization. Proceedings of the National Academy of Sciences of the United States of America. 1992;**89**(12):5321-5325

[20] Iqbal N, Iqbal N. Human Epidermal Growth Factor Receptor 2 (HER2) in cancers: Overexpression and therapeutic implications. Molecular Biology International. 2014; **852748**:2014

[21] Hubbard SR, Till JH. Protein tyrosine kinase structure and function. Annual Review of Biochemistry. 2000;**69**:373-398

[22] Carpenter G. Receptors for epidermal growth factor and other polypeptide mitogens. Annual Review of Biochemistry. 1987;**56**:881-914

[23] Roskoski R Jr. ErbB/HER protein-tyrosine kinases: Structures and small molecule inhibitors. Pharmacological Research. 2014;**87**:42-59

[24] Sierke SL, Cheng K, Kim HH, Koland JG. Biochemical characterization of the protein tyrosine kinase homology domain of the ErbB3 (HER3) receptor protein. The Biochemical Journal. 1997;**322**(Pt 3):757-763

[25] Kim HH, Vijapurkar U, Hellyer NJ, Bravo D, Koland JG. Signal transduction by epidermal growth factor and heregulin via the kinase-deficient ErbB3 protein. The Biochemical Journal. 1998;**334**(Pt 1):189-195

[26] Carrera AC, Alexandrov K, Roberts TM. The conserved lysine of the catalytic domain of protein kinases is actively involved in the phosphotransfer reaction and not required for anchoring ATP. Proceedings of the National Academy of Sciences of the United States of America. 1993;**90**(2):442-446

[27] Lemmon MA, Schlessinger J. Cell signaling by receptor tyrosine kinases. Cell. 2010;**141**(7):1117-1134

[28] Zaczek A, Brandt B, Bielawski KP. The diverse signaling network of EGFR, HER2, HER3 and HER4 tyrosine kinase receptors and the consequences for therapeutic approaches. Histology and Histopathology. 2005;**20**(3):1005-1015

[29] Wilson KJ, Gilmore JL, Foley J, Lemmon MA, Riese DJ 2nd. Functional selectivity of EGF family peptide growth factors: Implications for cancer. Pharmacology & Therapeutics. 2009;**122**(1):1-8

[30] Rubin I, Yarden Y. The basic biology of HER2. Annals of Oncology: Official Journal of the European Society for Medical Oncology. 2001;**12**(Suppl 1):S3-S8

[31] Burgess AW, Cho HS, Eigenbrot C, Ferguson KM, Garrett TP, Leahy DJ, et al. An open-and-shut case? Recent insights into the activation of EGF/ErbB receptors. Molecular Cell. 2003;**12**(3):541-552

[32] Sliwkowski MX. Ready to partner. Nature Structural Biology. 2003;**10**(3):158-159

[33] Chen H, Xu CF, Ma J, Eliseenkova AV, Li W, Pollock PM, et al. A crystallographic snapshot of tyrosine trans-phosphorylation in action. Proceedings of the National Academy of Sciences of the United States of America. 2008;**105**(50):19660-19665

[34] Paul MK, Mukhopadhyay AK. Tyrosine kinase—Role and significance in Cancer. International Journal of Medical Sciences. 2004;**1**(2):101-115

[35] Moasser MM. The oncogene HER2: Its signaling and transforming functions and its role in human cancer pathogenesis. Oncogene. 2007;**26**(45):6469-6487

[36] Nguyen B, Keane MM, Johnston PG. The biology of growth regulation in normal and malignant breast epithelium: From bench to clinic. Critical Reviews in Oncology/Hematology. 1995;**20**(3):223-236

[37] Hemmings BA, Restuccia DF. PI3K-PKB/Akt pathway. Cold Spring Harbor Perspectives in Biology. 2012;**4**(9):a011189

[38] Santarpia L, Lippman SM, El-Naggar AK. Targeting the MAPK-RAS-RAF signaling pathway in cancer therapy. Expert Opinion on Therapeutic Targets. 2012;**16**(1):103-119

[39] Baulida J, Kraus MH, Alimandi M, Di Fiore PP, Carpenter G. All ErbB receptors other than the epidermal growth factor receptor are endocytosis impaired. The Journal of Biological Chemistry. 1996;**271**(9):5251-5257

[40] Bertelsen V, Stang E. The mysterious ways of ErbB2/HER2 trafficking. Membranes. 2014; **4**(3):424-446

[41] Tzahar E, Waterman H, Chen X, Levkowitz G, Karunagaran D, Lavi S, et al. A hierarchical network of interreceptor interactions determines signal transduction by Neu differentiation factor/neuregulin and epidermal growth factor. Molecular and Cellular Biology. 1996;**16**(10):5276-5287

[42] Atalay G, Cardoso F, Awada A, Piccart MJ. Novel therapeutic strategies targeting the epidermal growth factor receptor (EGFR) family and its downstream effectors in breast cancer. Annals of Oncology: Official Journal of the European Society for Medical Oncology. 2003;**14**(9):1346-1363

[43] Graus-Porta D, Beerli RR, Daly JM, Hynes NE. ErbB-2, the preferred heterodimerization partner of all ErbB receptors, is a mediator of lateral signaling. The EMBO Journal. 1997;**16**(7):1647-1655

[44] Gutierrez C, Schiff R. HER2: Biology, detection, and clinical implications. Archives of Pathology & Laboratory Medicine. 2011;**135**(1):55-62

[45] Way TD, Lin JK. Role of HER2/HER3 co-receptor in breast carcinogenesis. Future Oncology. 2005;**1**(6):841-849

[46] Nahta R, Yuan LX, Zhang B, Kobayashi R, Esteva FJ. Insulin-like growth factor-I receptor/human epidermal growth factor receptor 2 heterodimerization contributes to trastuzumab resistance of breast cancer cells. Cancer Research. 2005;**65**(23):11118-11128

[47] Bononi A, Agnoletto C, De Marchi E, Marchi S, Patergnani S, Bonora M, et al. Protein kinases and phosphatases in the control of cell fate. Enzyme Research. 2011;**2011**:329098

[48] Arteaga CL. Epidermal growth factor receptor dependence in human tumors: More than just expression? The Oncologist. 2002;**7**(Suppl 4):31-39

[49] Brooks AN, Kilgour E, Smith PD. Molecular pathways: Fibroblast growth factor signaling: A new therapeutic opportunity in cancer. Clinical Cancer Research: An Official Journal of the American Association for Cancer Research. 2012;**18**(7):1855-1862

[50] Nishikawa R, Ji XD, Harmon RC, Lazar CS, Gill GN, Cavenee WK, et al. A mutant epidermal growth factor receptor common in human glioma confers enhanced tumorigenicity. Proceedings of the National Academy of Sciences of the United States of America. 1994;**91**(16):7727-7731

[51] Ocana A, Vera-Badillo F, Seruga B, Templeton A, Pandiella A, Amir E. HER3 overexpression and survival in solid tumors: A meta-analysis. Journal of the National Cancer Institute. 2013;**105**(4):266-273

[52] Roskoski R Jr. Vascular endothelial growth factor (VEGF) signaling in tumor progression. Critical Reviews in Oncology/Hematology. 2007;**62**(3):179-213

[53] Stern DF. Tyrosine kinase signalling in breast cancer: ErbB family receptor tyrosine kinases. Breast Cancer Research: BCR. 2000;**2**(3):176-183

[54] Hendriks BS, Opresko LK, Wiley HS, Lauffenburger D. Quantitative analysis of HER2-mediated effects on HER2 and epidermal growth factor receptor endocytosis: Distribution of homo- and heterodimers depends on relative HER2 levels. The Journal of Biological Chemistry. 2003;**278**(26):23343-23351

[55] Huang G, Chantry A, Epstein RJ. Overexpression of ErbB2 impairs ligand-dependent downregulation of epidermal growth factor receptors via a post-transcriptional mechanism. Journal of Cellular Biochemistry. 1999;**74**(1):23-30

[56] Wang Z, Zhang L, Yeung TK, Chen X. Endocytosis deficiency of epidermal growth factor (EGF) receptor-ErbB2 heterodimers in response to EGF stimulation. Molecular Biology of the Cell. 1999;**10**(5):1621-1636

[57] Lenferink AE, Pinkas-Kramarski R, van de Poll ML, van Vugt MJ, Klapper LN, Tzahar E, et al. Differential endocytic routing of homo- and hetero-dimeric ErbB tyrosine kinases confers signaling superiority to receptor heterodimers. The EMBO Journal. 1998;**17**(12): 3385-3397

[58] Waterman H, Yarden Y. Molecular mechanisms underlying endocytosis and sorting of ErbB receptor tyrosine kinases. FEBS Letters. 2001;**490**(3):142-152

[59] Hendriks BS, Wiley HS, Lauffenburger D. HER2-mediated effects on EGFR endosomal sorting: Analysis of biophysical mechanisms. Biophysical Journal. 2003;**85**(4):2732-2745

[60] Timms JF, White SL, O'Hare MJ, Waterfield MD. Effects of ErbB-2 overexpression on mitogenic signalling and cell cycle progression in human breast luminal epithelial cells. Oncogene. 2002;**21**(43):6573-6586

[61] Wolff AC, Hammond ME, Hicks DG, Dowsett M, McShane LM, Allison KH, et al. Recommendations for human epidermal growth factor receptor 2 testing in breast cancer: American Society of Clinical Oncology/College of American Pathologists clinical practice guideline update. Journal of Clinical Oncology: Official Journal of the American Society of Clinical Oncology. 2013;**31**(31):3997-4013

[62] Varshney D, Zhou YY, Geller SA, Alsabeh R. Determination of HER-2 status and chromosome 17 polysomy in breast carcinomas comparing HercepTest and PathVysion FISH assay. American Journal of Clinical Pathology. 2004;**121**(1):70-77

[63] Hanna W, Kahn HJ, Trudeau M. Evaluation of HER-2/neu (erbB-2) status in breast cancer: From bench to bedside. Modern Pathology: An Official Journal of the United States and Canadian Academy of Pathology, Inc. 1999;**12**(8):827-834

[64] Yildiz-Aktas IZ, Dabbs DJ, Bhargava R. The effect of cold ischemic time on the immuno-histochemical evaluation of estrogen receptor, progesterone receptor, and HER2 expression in invasive breast carcinoma. Modern Pathology: An Official Journal of the United States and Canadian Academy of Pathology, Inc. 2012;**25**(8):1098-1105

[65] Middleton LP, Price KM, Puig P, Heydon LJ, Tarco E, Sneige N, et al. Implementation of American Society of Clinical Oncology/College of American Pathologists HER2 Guideline Recommendations in a tertiary care facility increases HER2 immunohisto-chemistry and fluorescence in situ hybridization concordance and decreases the number of inconclusive cases. Archives of Pathology & Laboratory Medicine. 2009;**133**(5):775-780

[66] Tsuda H, Sasano H, Akiyama F, Kurosumi M, Hasegawa T, Osamura RY, et al. Evaluation of interobserver agreement in scoring immunohistochemical results of HER-2/neu (c-erbB-2) expression detected by HercepTest, Nichirei polyclonal antibody, CB11 and TAB250 in breast carcinoma. Pathology International. 2002;**52**(2):126-134

[67] Zhao J, Wu R, Au A, Marquez A, Yu Y, Shi Z. Determination of HER2 gene amplification by chromogenic in situ hybridization (CISH) in archival breast carcinoma. Modern Pathology: An Official Journal of the United States and Canadian Academy of Pathology, Inc. 2002;**15**(6):657-665

[68] Hoang MP, Sahin AA, Ordonez NG, Sneige N. HER-2/neu gene amplification compared with HER-2/neu protein overexpression and interobserver reproducibility in invasive breast carcinoma. American Journal of Clinical Pathology. 2000;**113**(6):852-859

[69] Sanderson MP, Dempsey PJ, Dunbar AJ. Control of ErbB signaling through metallopro-tease mediated ectodomain shedding of EGF-like factors. Growth Factors. 2006;**24**(2): 121-136

[70] Carney WP, Leitzel K, Ali S, Neumann R, Lipton A. HER-2/neu diagnostics in breast cancer. Breast Cancer Research: BCR. 2007;**9**(3):207

[71] Lam L, McAndrew N, Yee M, Fu T, Tchou JC, Zhang H. Challenges in the clinical utility of the serum test for HER2 ECD. Biochimica et Biophysica Acta. 2012;**1826**(1):199-208

[72] Moelans CB, de Weger RA, Van der Wall E, van Diest PJ. Current technologies for HER2 testing in breast cancer. Critical Reviews in Oncology/Hematology. 2011;**80**(3):380-392

[73] Hicks DG, Tubbs RR. Assessment of the HER2 status in breast cancer by fluorescence in situ hybridization: A technical review with interpretive guidelines. Human Pathology. 2005;**36**(3):250-261

[74] Ross JS, Slodkowska EA, Symmans WF, Pusztai L, Ravdin PM, Hortobagyi GN. The HER-2 receptor and breast cancer: Ten years of targeted anti-HER-2 therapy and person-alized medicine. The Oncologist. 2009;**14**(4):320-368

[75] Tse CH, Hwang HC, Goldstein LC, Kandalaft PL, Wiley JC, Kussick SJ, et al. Determining true HER2 gene status in breast cancers with polysomy by using alternative chromo-some 17 reference genes: Implications for anti-HER2 targeted therapy. Journal of Clinical Oncology: Official Journal of the American Society of Clinical Oncology. 2011; **29**(31):4168-4174

[76] Varga Z, Noske A, Ramach C, Padberg B, Moch H. Assessment of HER2 status in breast cancer: Overall positivity rate and accuracy by fluorescence in situ hybridization and immunohistochemistry in a single institution over 12 years: A quality control study. BMC Cancer. 2013;**13**:615

[77] Bartlett JM, Going JJ, Mallon EA, Watters AD, Reeves JR, Stanton P, et al. Evaluating HER2 amplification and overexpression in breast cancer. The Journal of Pathology. 2001;**195**(4):422-428

[78] Paik S, Bryant J, Tan-Chiu E, Romond E, Hiller W, Park K, et al. Real-world performance of HER2 testing--National Surgical Adjuvant Breast and bowel project experience. Journal of the National Cancer Institute. 2002;**94**(11):852-854

[79] Press MF, Hung G, Godolphin W, Slamon DJ. Sensitivity of HER-2/neu antibodies in archival tissue samples: Potential source of error in immunohistochemical studies of oncogene expression. Cancer Research. 1994;**54**(10):2771-2777

[80] Tubbs RR, Pettay JD, Roche PC, Stoler MH, Jenkins RB, Grogan TM. Discrepancies in clinical laboratory testing of eligibility for trastuzumab therapy: Apparent immunohistochemical false-positives do not get the message. Journal of Clinical Oncology: Official Journal of the American Society of Clinical Oncology. 2001;**19**(10):2714-2721

[81] Yeh IT. Measuring HER-2 in breast cancer. Immunohistochemistry, FISH, or ELISA? American Journal of Clinical Pathology. 2002;**117**(Suppl):S26-S35

[82] Bhargava R, Lal P, Chen B. Chromogenic in situ hybridization for the detection of HER-2/neu gene amplification in breast cancer with an emphasis on tumors with borderline and low-level amplification: Does it measure up to fluorescence in situ hybridization? American Journal of Clinical Pathology. 2005;**123**(2):237-243

[83] Yaziji H, Goldstein LC, Barry TS, Werling R, Hwang H, Ellis GK, et al. HER-2 testing in breast cancer using parallel tissue-based methods. Journal of the American Medical Association. 2004;**291**(16):1972-1977

[84] Ridolfi RL, Jamehdor MR, Arber JM. HER-2/neu testing in breast carcinoma: A combined immunohistochemical and fluorescence in situ hybridization approach. Modern Pathology: An Official Journal of the United States and Canadian Academy of Pathology, Inc. 2000;**13**(8):866-873

[85] Dowsett M, Hanna WM, Kockx M, Penault-Llorca F, Ruschoff J, Gutjahr T, et al. Standardization of HER2 testing: Results of an international proficiency-testing ring study. Modern Pathology: An Official Journal of the United States and Canadian Academy of Pathology, Inc. 2007;**20**(5):584-591

[86] Furrer D, Jacob S, Caron C, Sanschagrin F, Provencher L, Diorio C. Validation of a new classifier for the automated analysis of the human epidermal growth factor receptor 2 (HER2) gene amplification in breast cancer specimens. Diagnostic Pathology. 2013;**8**:17

[87] Stevens R, Almanaseer I, Gonzalez M, Caglar D, Knudson RA, Ketterling RP, et al. Analysis of HER2 gene amplification using an automated fluorescence in situ hybridization signal enumeration system. The Journal of Molecular Diagnostics: JMD. 2007;**9**(2):144-150

[88] Tubbs RR, Pettay JD, Swain E, Roche PC, Powell W, Hicks DG, et al. Automation of manual components and image quantification of direct dual label fluorescence in situ hybridization (FISH) for HER2 gene amplification: A feasibility study. Applied Immunohistochemistry & Molecular Morphology: AIMM. 2006;**14**(4):436-440

[89] Furrer D, Sanschagrin F, Jacob S, Diorio C. Advantages and disadvantages of technologies for HER2 testing in breast cancer specimens. American Journal of Clinical Pathology. 2015;**144**(5):686-703

[90] Penault-Llorca F, Bilous M, Dowsett M, Hanna W, Osamura RY, Ruschoff J, et al. Emerging technologies for assessing HER2 amplification. American Journal of Clinical Pathology. 2009;**132**(4):539-548

[91] Gong Y, Gilcrease M, Sneige N. Reliability of chromogenic in situ hybridization for detecting HER-2 gene status in breast cancer: Comparison with fluorescence in situ hybridization and assessment of interobserver reproducibility. Modern Pathology: An Official Journal of the United States and Canadian Academy of Pathology, Inc. 2005;**18**(8):1015-1021

[92] Isola J, Tanner M, Forsyth A, Cooke TG, Watters AD, Bartlett JM. Interlaboratory comparison of HER-2 oncogene amplification as detected by chromogenic and fluorescence in situ hybridization. Clinical Cancer Research: An Official Journal of the American Association for Cancer Research. 2004;**10**(14):4793-4798

[93] Gupta D, Middleton LP, Whitaker MJ, Abrams J. Comparison of fluorescence and chromogenic in situ hybridization for detection of HER-2/neu oncogene in breast cancer. American Journal of Clinical Pathology. 2003;**119**(3):381-387

[94] Garcia-Caballero T, Grabau D, Green AR, Gregory J, Schad A, Kohlwes E, et al. Determination of HER2 amplification in primary breast cancer using dual-colour chromogenic in situ hybridization is comparable to fluorescence in situ hybridization: A European multicentre study involving 168 specimens. Histopathology. 2010;**56**(4):472-480

[95] Lambros MB, Natrajan R, Reis-Filho JS. Chromogenic and fluorescent in situ hybridization in breast cancer. Human Pathology. 2007;**38**(8):1105-1122

[96] Hwang CC, Pintye M, Chang LC, Chen HY, Yeh KY, Chein HP, et al. Dual-colour chromogenic in-situ hybridization is a potential alternative to fluorescence in-situ hybridization in HER2 testing. Histopathology. 2011;**59**(5):984-992

[97] Powell RD, Pettay JD, Powell WC, Roche PC, Grogan TM, Hainfeld JF, et al. Metallographic in situ hybridization. Human Pathology. 2007;**38**(8):1145-1159

[98] Bartlett JM, Campbell FM, Ibrahim M, Wencyk P, Ellis I, Kay E, et al. Chromogenic in situ hybridization: A multicenter study comparing silver in situ hybridization with FISH. American Journal of Clinical Pathology. 2009;**132**(4):514-520

[99] Francis GD, Jones MA, Beadle GF, Stein SR. Bright-field in situ hybridization for HER2 gene amplification in breast cancer using tissue microarrays: Correlation between chromogenic (CISH) and automated silver-enhanced (SISH) methods with patient outcome. Diagnostic Molecular Pathology: The American Journal of Surgical Pathology, Part B. 2009;**18**(2):88-95

[100] Nitta H, Hauss-Wegrzyniak B, Lehrkamp M, Murillo AE, Gaire F, Farrell M, et al. Development of automated brightfield double in situ hybridization (BDISH) application for HER2 gene and chromosome 17 centromere (CEN 17) for breast carcinomas and an assay performance comparison to manual dual color HER2 fluorescence in situ hybridization (FISH). Diagnostic Pathology. 2008;**3**:41

[101] Schiavon BN, Jasani B, de Brot L, Vassallo J, Damascena A, Cirullo-Neto J, et al. Evaluation of reliability of FISH versus brightfield dual-probe in situ hybridization (BDISH) for frontline assessment of HER2 status in breast cancer samples in a community setting: Influence of poor tissue preservation. The American Journal of Surgical Pathology. 2012;**36**(10):1489-1496

[102] Bartlett JM, Campbell FM, Ibrahim M, O'Grady A, Kay E, Faulkes C, et al. A UK NEQAS ISH multicenter ring study using the Ventana HER2 dual-color ISH assay. American Journal of Clinical Pathology. 2011;**135**(1):157-162

[103] Franchet C, Filleron T, Cayre A, Mounie E, Penault-Llorca F, Jacquemier J, et al. Instant-quality fluorescence in-situ hybridization as a new tool for HER2 testing in breast cancer: A comparative study. Histopathology. 2014;**64**(2):274-283

[104] Matthiesen SH, Hansen CM. Fast and non-toxic in situ hybridization without blocking of repetitive sequences. PLoS One. 2012;**7**(7):e40675

[105] Ohlschlegel C, Kradolfer D, Hell M, Jochum W. Comparison of automated and manual FISH for evaluation of HER2 gene status on breast carcinoma core biopsies. BMC Clinical Pathology. 2013;**13**:13

[106] Cronin M, Pho M, Dutta D, Stephans JC, Shak S, Kiefer MC, et al. Measurement of gene expression in archival paraffin-embedded tissues: Development and performance of a 92-gene reverse transcriptase-polymerase chain reaction assay. The American Journal of Pathology. 2004;**164**(1):35-42

[107] Noske A, Loibl S, Darb-Esfahani S, Roller M, Kronenwett R, Muller BM, et al. Comparison of different approaches for assessment of HER2 expression on protein and mRNA level: Prediction of chemotherapy response in the neoadjuvant GeparTrio trial (NCT00544765). Breast Cancer Research and Treatment. 2011;**126**(1):109-117

[108] Jacquemier J, Spyratos F, Esterni B, Mozziconacci MJ, Antoine M, Arnould L, et al. SISH/CISH or qPCR as alternative techniques to FISH for determination of HER2 amplification status on breast tumors core needle biopsies: A multicenter experience based on 840 cases. BMC Cancer. 2013;**13**:351

[109] Merkelbach-Bruse S, Wardelmann E, Behrens P, Losen I, Buettner R, Friedrichs N. Current diagnostic methods of HER-2/neu detection in breast cancer with special regard to real-time PCR. The American Journal of Surgical Pathology. 2003;**27**(12):1565-1570

[110] Nistor A, Watson PH, Pettigrew N, Tabiti K, Dawson A, Myal Y. Real-time PCR complements immunohistochemistry in the determination of HER-2/neu status in breast cancer. BMC Clinical Pathology. 2006;**6**:2

[111] Esteva FJ, Yu D, Hung MC, Hortobagyi GN. Molecular predictors of response to trastuzumab and lapatinib in breast cancer. Nature Reviews Clinical Oncology. 2010;**7**(2):98-107

Chapter 3

Is Melanoma a Hormone-Dependent Cancer or a Hormone-Responsive Cancer?

Pandurangan Ramaraj

Additional information is available at the end of the chapter

http://dx.doi.org/10.5772/intechopen.76499

Abstract

Melanoma, a potentially fatal form of skin cancer is on the rise. This review not only underlines the close connection between skin and endocrine system, but also lists evidences from multiple sources epidemiological, clinical, previous in vivo and in vitro studies regarding the involvement of sex steroids in melanoma. Incidentally, clinical studies underscored the involvement of sex steroids in the protective function in melanoma in menstruating females. But, none of these studies identified the sex steroids involved in the protective function in melanoma in menstruating females. The sex steroid involved in this innate protection in melanoma in menstruating females has not been investigated by scientists, though advances have been made in immunotherapy with accompanying side effects. In this context, our in vitro studies on mouse and human melanoma cell lines, along with literature survey, pointed to progesterone as the possible female sex steroid involved in the protective function in melanoma. Based on our findings and previous studies, it is concluded in this review that melanoma is not a hormone-dependent cancer. But, it may be a hormone-sensitive or responsive cancer, as hormones (sex steroids) inhibited melanoma cell proliferation in vitro. This new understanding will help in developing new therapy or target for melanoma treatment.

Keywords: melanoma, epidemiological studies, clinical studies, in vivo and in vitro studies, protective function, progesterone, hormone-responsive cancer

1. Introduction

The question that has been raised over the years, whether melanoma is a hormone-dependent cancer or not still lacks a clear-cut answer [1–4]. However, in this review, an attempt has been made to collect evidences from multiple sources to point out the nature of melanoma. Melanoma, the fatal form of skin cancer accounts for less than 2% of skin cancer, but it is

IntechOpen

responsible for 75% of deaths due to skin cancer [5]. According to the American Cancer Society reports known as Cancer Statistics, melanoma is on the rise. In 2018, in the United States, 91,270 new cases will be diagnosed with an estimated 9320 deaths [6]. Melanoma occurs mostly on the skin [7]; however, some rare forms of melanoma can occur in other areas such as cornea, uvea, and gastrointestinal tract [7]. Epidemiological data indicated an increased mortality rates in males than in females [8], suggesting a sex difference. Clinical studies showed that menstruating females were better protected (delayed metastasis and increased survival) in melanoma than postmenopausal women and men of any age [9], clearly indicating the role of sex steroid hormones in the protection function. It is important to point out that skin itself functions as an endocrine organ [10], even though it is not acknowledged as one. Skin possesses many of the enzymes necessary for synthesis of steroid hormones [11]. In fact, most of the peripheral conversions of dehydroenpiandrosterone (DHEA) and androstenedione (AD) to testosterone and estradiol take place in the skin [12]. This area of endocrinology is known as intracrinology [12]. In addition, skin is also a target organ for various hormones. Sex steroids such as androgens, estrogens, and progestins are essential for a healthy skin [13]. Melanocyte, which is transformed to melanoma cell is also under the influence of melanocyte-stimulating hormone (MSH) from pituitary [14]. Hence, it is natural to ask the question whether melanoma is a hormone-dependent cancer like breast, prostate, and endometrial cancers. Generally, melanoma is not labeled as a hormone-dependent cancer because of the belief that UV rays from the Sun is the major cause for melanoma [15]. UV rays cause DNA damages and other inflammatory changes in the skin, which result in skin cancer. About 90% of melanoma is caused by environmental factors such as UV rays, radiations, and only 10% is inherited in the family. So, melanoma is never considered as a hormone-dependent cancer. However, existing evidences point to a hormone relatedness or a hormone-responsive nature of melanoma cancer:

1. Evidences of relationship between skin and endocrine system: there is a close connection between skin and endocrine system, as shown by the following examples.

   a. All the components of a functional hypothalamo-pituitary-adrenal axis analog are present in the skin.

   b. Presence of enzymes involved in steroid hormone synthesis in skin cells: the level of local steroid production depends on the expression of androgen- and estrogen-synthesizing enzymes present in specific cell types. Five major enzymes are involved in the activation and deactivation of androgens in the skin [13].

   c. Actions of sex steroid hormones on skin: skin is a target organ for sex steroid hormones. Androgens are essential for differentiation and growth of Sebocyte and hair growth. Estrogen is responsible for skin pigmentation and skin cancer. Progesterone functions, though not clear is essential for treating acne [13].

   d. Endocrine disorders manifested on the skin:

      i. Association of insulin resistance and metabolic syndrome with acne: post-adolescent male patients with acne more commonly have insulin resistance [16]. This resistance may be a stage of prediabetes and the patients may develop hyperinsulinemia or type 2 diabetes in the future.

ii. Association of cutaneous findings and systemic abnormalities in women suspected of having polycystic ovary syndrome (PCOS): Hirsutism and acne are the most reliable cutaneous markers of PCOS and require a comprehensive skin examination to diagnose [17].

iii. Psoriasis severity may influence type 2 diabetes risk: people living with psoriasis are not only at higher risk of type 2 diabetes, but their risk also rises in line with the skin disease's severity [18].

It is evident from the above mentioned examples that skin is not only an endocrine organ which produces various hormones, but also has a close relationship with systemic endocrine system.

2. Evidences from epidemiological data

According to the epidemiological SEER data [8] known as Surveillance, Epidemiology and End Results program, a database maintained by NCI, there has been an increase in the incidence of melanoma. The incidence of melanoma ('03-'07) for men and women were 26.7 per 100,000 and 16.7 per 100,000 respectively. There has been an increase in death rate also. Even in the death rate, there was a difference between males and females. The mortality rate for males was 4.0 per 100,000, whereas for females it was 1.7 per 100,000. Males have increased mortality rate than females. Death rate was cut more than half in females. Similarly, malignant melanoma database (1971–2012) maintained by UK Cancer Research Council [19] also showed that the morality rate was higher in males than in females over the years. The data [20] was almost similar from Australian continent, where the incidence of melanoma is the highest in the world. From 1982 to 2016, the number of melanoma diagnosed in Australia increased from 3526 to an estimated 13,280. The age-standardized incidence rate increased for both males and females, from 28 to 60 cases per 100,000 males, and from 26 to 39 cases per 100,000 females. Data showed males were more prone to melanoma than females [20]. Thus epidemiological data from three continents clearly showed that males were more affected by melanoma than females. These gender differences in melanoma demand an investigation of the effect of sex hormones on this malignancy.

3. Evidences from clinical studies

Clinical studies supported the epidemiological findings. Clinical studies showed that menstruating females were better protected (delayed metastasis and increased survival) in melanoma than post-menopausal women and men of any ages [9]. This very difference between menstruating females and postmenopausal women clearly indicated the involvement of steroid hormones in protecting menstruating females in melanoma. However, these data base were not correlated with the steroid status of females. Studies published between 1977 and 1966 showed women had better survival in all but 4 out of 22 epidemiologic studies [21]. Two female hormones could be involved in rendering protection, namely estrogen and progesterone. First, estrogen as the hormone protecting menstruating females in melanoma: estrogen receptor antagonist tamoxifen was evaluated as a single agent in 12 studies covering 213 patients with metastatic melanoma cancer [22]; the response rate was only 7%. Moreover, estrogen receptors were found in some cancers only by biochemical and histochemical tests but not by the immunohistochemical tests using monoclonal antibodies [23]. Second, progesterone as the possible female sex hormone involved in the protection: there were only limited in vitro studies [24, 25] and they were also not tied to the protective function in melanoma. According to the data published on pregnancy and melanoma, several studies reported statistically no significant differences in survival rates between controls (non-pregnant women with malignant melanoma) and women diagnosed with melanoma stage I or II during pregnancy [26–28]. Studies also found no association between melanoma and oral contraceptives [29, 30]. Data on the relationship between melanoma and hormone replacement therapy were meager and it seemed that exogenous hormones did not influence the risk for malignant melanoma [31, 32]. So, clinical studies underlined the involvement of female sex steroid hormones in protecting menstruating females in melanoma. But, these clinical studies did not identify the exact female hormone involved in the protection.

4. Evidences from animal studies

Animal studies also showed the involvement of sex steroid hormones in the regulation of melanoma growth and there were also differences in the regulation of melanoma growth between male and female mice.

a. Female survival benefit with metastatic melanoma was observed, when melanoma cells produced liver metastases preferentially in male compared to female mice [33].

b. In another study, estrogen receptor-positive human melanomas cells grew more slowly in females than in males mice [34].

c. Similarly, dihydrotestosterone was shown to stimulate proliferation. But, in a follow-up study, male mice transplanted with melanoma showed increased survival after treatment with anti-androgen receptor hydroxyflutamide [35].

d. Male mice were significantly more susceptible to carcinogen-induced skin cancer than female mice [36].

e. Similarly male mice were more susceptible to UV-B induced skin carcinogenesis than female mice [37]

f. Research work presented in one study showed that metapristone (a metabolite of mifepristone (RU-486)) had a remarkable effect of preventing cancer metastasis of B16-F10 cells in vivo compared with mifepristone [38].

5. Evidences from previous cell-culture studies

Apart from epidemiological, clinical, and in vivo animal studies, various in vitro studies using a variety of melanoma cell lines showed the inhibitory effect of steroid hormones on melanoma cell growth, suggesting melanoma could be a hormone-sensitive or responsive cancer.

a. In one study, 2-methoxyestradiol (2-ME), an estrogenic metabolite inhibited the growth of all melanoma cells tested, without inhibiting the growth of non-tumorigenic cells [39].

b. Data from another study suggested that 17-β-estradiol, progesterone, and dihydrotestosterone suppressed the growth of melanoma cells by inhibiting interleukin-8 production in a receptor-dependent manner [25].

c. However, Feucht et al. investigated three human melanoma cell lines and found no effect either by estradiol or tamoxifen on melanoma cell growth in vitro [34].

d. Another in vitro study indicated a direct inhibitory effect of testosterone on growth of an amelanotic strain which in vivo grew faster in female hamsters [40].

e. The findings in another study indicated that glucocorticoids exerted some influence on the growth of human melanoma cells and this effect was mediated through glucocorticoid receptor [41].

f. Only study which showed a stimulatory effect was with melanocyte, where α-MSH stimulated melanocyte proliferation in a dose-dependent manner, but its stimulatory effect required bFGF and/or the activation of protein kinase C [42].

g. Another in vitro study showed that melatonin at physiological concentrations (1 nM to 10 pM) inhibited metastatic mouse melanoma (B16BL6) cell growth [43].

6. Evidences from our studies on mouse melanoma (B16F10) cell line

a. Progesterone effect on mouse melanoma (B16F10) cell growth: based on previous research work and literature survey, initially four sex steroids were checked for their effect on mouse melanoma (B16F10) cell growth [44]. Of the four steroids checked [dehydroepiandrosterone (DHEA), androstenedione (AD), testosterone (T) and progesterone (P)], progesterone showed significant inhibition (87%) of mouse melanoma cell growth. Though other steroid hormones also showed inhibition of cell growth, but it was not as significant as that of progesterone inhibition (**Figure 1**).

b. Progesterone dose-response study with mouse melanoma cells: as the initial experiment was carried out at high concentrations (100, 150, 200 μM) of hormones, a follow-up dose-response study was carried out with progesterone alone. Dose-curve study with progesterone showed a dose-dependent decrease in mouse melanoma cell growth (**Figure 2**).

c. Further studies with mouse melanoma cell line: further studies (data not shown) showed that the effect of progesterone on mouse melanoma cells was not a toxic, not a spurious or not a non-specific effect [44]. The only other steroid which showed a significant inhibition of mouse melanoma cell growth was progesterone-receptor antagonist RU-486, a synthetic steroid (**Figure 3**).

d. Mechanism of progesterone action on mouse melanoma cell line: since RU-486 also showed a dose-dependent inhibition of mouse melanoma cell growth, it was decided to find out whether the actions of progesterone and RU-486 were mediated through progesterone receptor. A co-incubation study was carried out with fixed concentration of progesterone (50 µM) and varying concentrations of RU-486 (10, 50, 100 µM). Co-incubation study showed an additive effect (data not shown) on mouse melanoma cell growth suggesting that the action was not mediated through progesterone receptor [44].

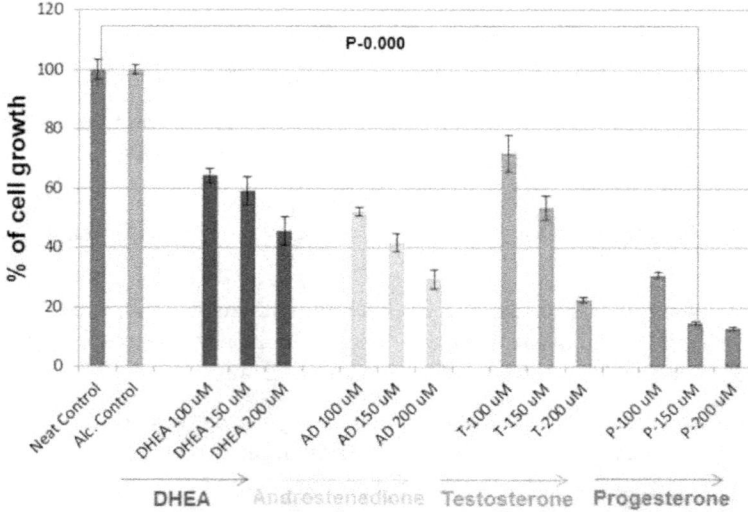

Figure 1. Various steroid hormones effect on mouse melanoma (B16F10) cell growth: three androgens (DHEA, AD, T) and one female sex steroid hormone (P) were checked for their effect on mouse melanoma cell growth at 100, 150, and 200 µM concentrations. Cells were incubated with the hormones separately for 48 h. After 48 h, cell growth was assessed by MTT assay. All the steroids checked showed dose-dependent decrease in cell growth. But, progesterone showed a significant inhibition of cell growth (87%) at 200 µM concentration.

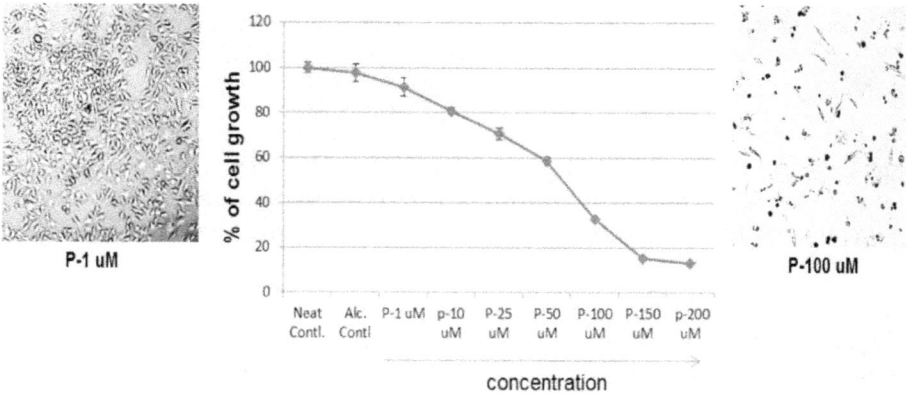

Figure 2. Dose-response study with mouse melanoma cell line: since the initial study was carried out at high concentrations, a dose-response study was carried out with progesterone starting from 1 to 200 µM. Progesterone showed a dose-dependent decrease in mouse melanoma cell growth with significant inhibition at 200 µM concentration. Cell growth was monitored by 3-(4,5-dimethylthiazol-2-yl)-2,5-diphenyltetrazolium bromide (MTT) assay.

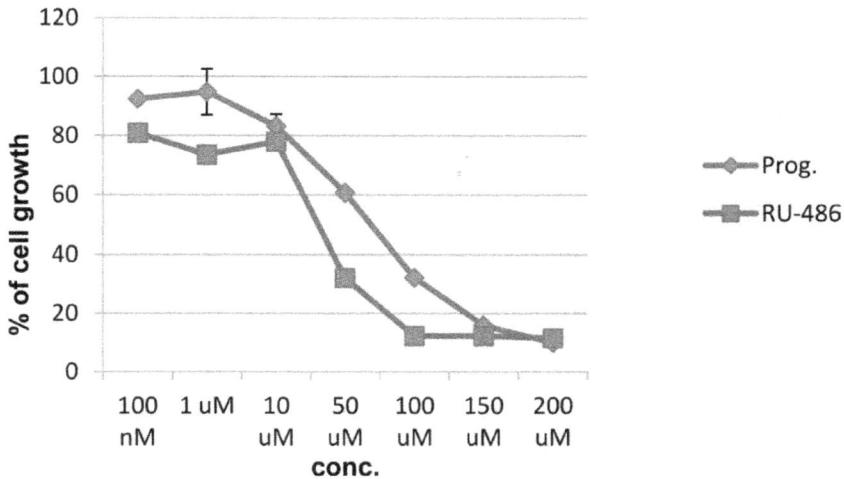

Figure 3. Comparison of dose-response curves of progesterone and RU-486: both progesterone and RU-486 were treated separately for 48 h. After 48 h, cell growth was assessed by MTT assay. Dose-response curve of RU-486 was compared with that of progesterone. The dose–response curves were very similar to each other.

7. Evidences from our studies on human melanoma (BLM) cell line

a. Dose-response study with progesterone and RU-486 on human melanoma cell line: the sex steroids (progesterone and RU-486), which showed inhibition on mouse cell line were checked on human melanoma (BLM) cell line for their effect [45, 46]. Progesterone and RU-486 also showed a dose-dependent inhibition of human melanoma cell growth (**Figure 4**).

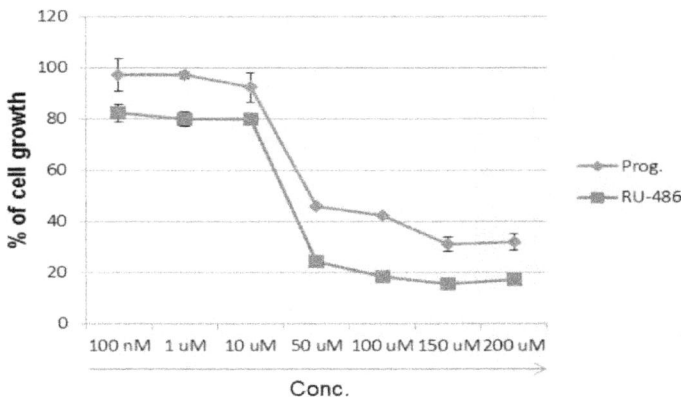

Figure 4. Dose-response study of progesterone and RU-486 on human melanoma cell line: progesterone and RU-486 were incubated separately with human melanoma cells for 48 h. After 48 h of incubation, cell growth was measured by MTT assay. Dose-response study of both progesterone and RU-486 showed a dose-dependent decrease of human melanoma cell growth.

b. Mechanism of action of progesterone on human melanoma cells: since progesterone and RU-486 separately showed a dose-dependent inhibition of human melanoma cell growth, it was decided to find out whether these actions were mediated through progesterone receptor on human melanoma cell line. Therefore, co-incubation study, just like the one on mouse melanoma cell line was carried out. Co-incubation study showed that the effect was not mediated through progesterone receptor (**Figure 5**). In fact, co-incubation of the two steroids (progesterone and RU-486) showed an additive effect on cell growth inhibition, suggesting the actions were mediated through two different mechanisms.

c. Mechanism of inhibition of human melanoma cell growth by progesterone: since the co-incubation study suggested that the mechanism of action of progesterone and RU-486 could be different, it was decided to find out the mechanism of inhibition of human melanoma cell growth by progesterone. After having ruled out necrosis and apoptosis as the mechanism of inhibition of cell growth, it was found out that autophagy was the cause for cell growth inhibition by co-incubating progesterone and 3-methyl adenine (3-MA) on melanoma cells. 3-methyl adenine (3-MA) had been used in various studies to check or

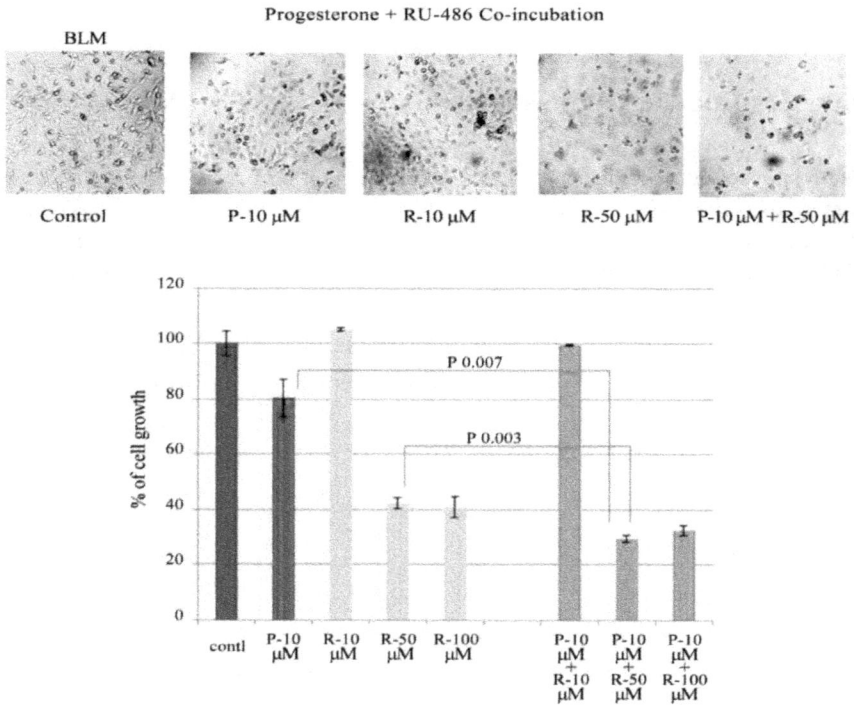

Figure 5. Co-incubation of progesterone and RU-486: a fixed concentration of progesterone (10 μM) was co-incubated with varying concentrations of RU-486 (10, 50, 100 μM). Co-incubated cells showed an additive effect on cell growth inhibition, suggesting the action was mediated through different mechanisms and not through progesterone receptor.

inhibit autophagy [47–49]. Therefore, the mechanism of inhibition of human melanoma cell growth by progesterone was due to autophagy (**Figure 6**).

d. Suppression of adhesion and migration functions of human melanoma cells by progesterone: metastasis of cancer involves adhesion, migration, and invasion functions. Progesterone ability to suppress metastasis was checked by in vitro adhesion and migration assays after treatment with progesterone for 48 h [50]. Progesterone at 100-µM concentration decreased adhesion function to 71% compared to untreated control cells at 100%. Similarly progesterone at 50 µM significantly decreased migration to 20% compared to untreated control cells at 100%. Adhesion and migration assays suggested that progesterone could be playing a role in delayed metastasis, as reported in clinical studies [9] (**Figure 7**).

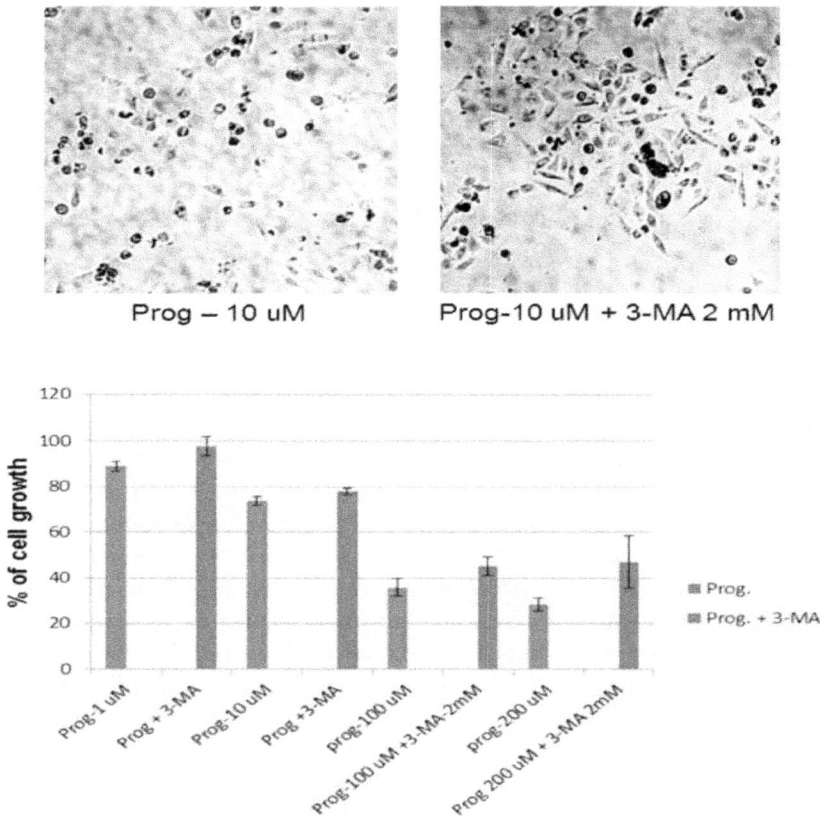

Prog – 10 uM   Prog-10 uM + 3-MA 2 mM

Figure 6. Mechanism of human melanoma (BLM) cell growth inhibition by progesterone: after having ruled out necrosis and apoptosis as mechanism of inhibition, it was decided to find out whether autophagy was the mechanism of inhibition of cell growth. So, cells were co-incubated with progesterone and 3-MA (2 mM) for 48 h. After 48 h, cell growth was monitored by MTT assay. 3-methyl adenine (3-MA) partially rescued melanoma cell growth, showing a slight increase in co-incubated cell growth compared to progesterone alone treated cell growth. 3-methyl adenine (3-MA) had been shown to disrupt the formation of autophagsome/lysosomal degradation in various studies [47–49].

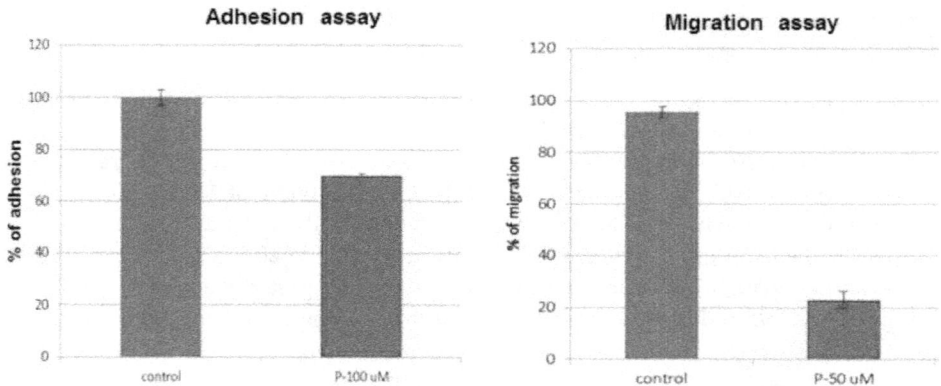

Figure 7. Suppression of adhesion and migration functions by progesterone: human melanoma cells were treated with progesterone for 48 h in petri dishes. After 48 h, cells were harvested from control and progesterone treated cells. Adhesion assay was carried out in a 96 well plate with 30,000 cells/wells. Cells were incubated for 60 min and washed. Cells attached to the plate were fixed with 2% paraformaldehyde and stained with 0.2% crystal violet dye. Purple color dye was eluted with isopropanol and assayed at 570 nm in a plate reader. For migration assay, treated cells were placed in a 24 well plate and allowed to become confluent. Cells were scratched in the middle of the plate with a tip, which was considered as 0 time point and cells were allowed to incubate for 24 h. After 24 h, percentage of cells migrated to the cleared space was calculated with a software.

8. Summary

There is a close connection between skin and endocrine system, as shown by the neuroen-docrine properties of skin. Skin not only functions as an endocrine organ but also as a target organ for various hormones. Epidemiological studies highlighted the differences in mortal-ity rate between males and females and hinted the involvement of hormones in melanoma. Clinical studies pinpointed the role of sex steroids, mainly female sex steroids, in melanoma. Animal studies also highlighted the involvement of sex steroids in melanoma. In vitro studies with steroid hormones showed inhibition of melanoma cell growth. Our studies showed the in vitro effect of progesterone on mouse and human melanoma cell growth. In our studies, progesterone showed significant inhibition of mouse and human melanoma cell growth. The mechanism of inhibition was due to autophagy and the effect was not mediated through pro-gesterone receptor. In vitro study also showed suppression of adhesion and migration func-tions after progesterone treatment, suggesting progesterone could be involved in delayed metastasis of cancer. This in vitro finding supported the clinical studies which showed men-struating females (whose progesterone level vary between 1000 and 1500 ng/dL) were bet-ter protected in melanoma than post-menopausal women (whose progesterone level vary between 20 and 100 ng/dL) and men of any age. A similar study with different human mela-noma (A375, A875) cell lines by Fang et al. [51] also showed that progesterone and RU-486 inhibited melanoma cell growth and this effect was also not mediated through progesterone receptor. Similar result was observed in another study using progesterone and the same mela-noma cell lines by Moroni et al. [31]. Kanda and Watanbe [25] had already shown the inhibi-tion of human melanoma cells by progesterone. Thus the inhibition of melanoma cell growth by progesterone was observed by 3 other different groups. Thus, the preceding studies, our own studies, and previous studies by others lend support to the idea that melanoma is amenable to hormone action and that melanoma is sensitive or responsive to steroid hormones.

9. Conclusion

Evidences from multiple sources (epidemiological, clinical, in vivo, and in vitro) suggested the involvement of hormones in melanoma and that melanoma was amenable to hormone action. But, unlike breast, ovary, and prostate cancers, addition of hormones did not stimulate proliferation of melanoma cells, suggesting melanoma was not a hormone-dependent cancer. However, addition of hormones suppressed melanoma cell proliferation, suggesting melanoma might be a hormone-sensitive or responsive cancer. Therefore, acquisition of melanoma may not be hormone dependent, but survival (suppression of cancer cell proliferation) in melanoma may be hormone dependent. Hence, based on epidemiological findings, clinical studies, literature reports of previous in vivo and in vitro experiments, and our own experiments, melanoma may be considered as a hormone-sensitive or responsive cancer. This understanding will help in generating new therapy or therapeutic target for melanoma treatment.

Declaration of interest

Author has nothing to declare.

Author details

Pandurangan Ramaraj

Address all correspondence to: pramaraj@atsu.edu

Department of Biochemistry, Kirksville College of Osteopathic Medicine, A.T. Still University, Kirksville, MO, USA

References

[1] Sadoff L, Winkley J, Tyson S. Is malignant melanoma an endocrine-dependent tumor? Oncology. 1973;**27**:244-257

[2] Gupta A, Driscoll MS. Do hormones influence melanoma? Facts and controversies. Clinics in Dermatology. 2010;**28**(3):287-292

[3] De Giorgi V, Gori A, Alfaioli B, Papi F, Grazzini M, Rossari S, Lotti T, Massi D. Influence of sex hormones on melanoma. Journal of Clinical Oncology. 2011;**29**(4):e94-e95

[4]   Mitkov M, Joseph R, Coplane J 3rd. Steroid hormone influence on melanomagenesis. Molecular and Cellular Endocrinology. 2015;**417**:94-102. DOI: 10.1016/j.mce.2015.09.020

[5]   Gray-Schopfer V, Wellbrock C, Marais R. Melanoma biology and new targeted therapy. Nature. 2007;**445**:851-857

[6]   Siegel RL, Miller KD, Jemal A. Cancer statistics. CA: A Cancer Journal for Clinicians. 2018;**68**:7-30. DOI: 10.3322/caac.21442

[7]   https://www.cancer.org/cancer/melanoma-skin-cancer.html

[8]   http://seer.cancer.gov/statfacts/html/melan.html

[9]   Kemeny MM, Busch E, Stewart AK, Mench HR. Superior survival of young women with malignant melanoma. American Journal of Surgery. 1988;**175**:437-444

[10] Zouboulis CC. Human skin: An independent peripheral endocrine organ. Hormone Research. 2000;**54**:230-242

[11] Zouboulis CC. The human skin as a hormone target and an endocrine gland. Hormones. 2004;**3**(1):9-26

[12] Labrie F. DHEA and its transformation into androgens and estrogens in peripheral target tissues: Intracrinology. Frontieres in Euroendocrinology. 2001;**22**(3):185-212

[13] Zouboulis CC, Chen WC, Thornton MJ, Qin K, Rosenfield R. Sexual hormones in human skin. Hormone and Metabolic Research. 2007;**39**(2):85-95

[14] Ranson M, Posen S, Mason RS. Human melanocytes as a target tissue for hormones: In vitro studies with 1α-25 dihydroxy vitamin D$_3$, α-melanocyte stimulating hormone and β-estradiol. The Journal of Investigative Dermatology. 1988;**91**:593-598

[15] Rass K, Reicharth J. UV damage and DNA repair in malignant melanoma and non-melanoma skin cancer. Advances in Experimental Medicine and Biology. 2008;**624**:162-178. DOI: 10.1007/978-0-387-77574-6_13

[16] Nagpal M, De D, Handa S, Pal A, Sachdeva N. Insulin resistance and metabolic syndrome in young men with acne. JAMA Dermatology. 2016;**152**(4):399-404. DOI: 10.1001/jamadermatol.2015.4499

[17] Schmidt TH, Khanijow K, Cedars MI, Huddleston H, Pasch L, Wang ET, Lee J, Zane LT, Shinkai K. Cutaneous findings and systemic associations in women with polycystic ovary syndrome. JAMA Dermatology. 2016;**152**(4):391-398. DOI: 10.1001/jama dermatol.2015.4498

[18] Wan MT, Shin DB, Hubbard RA, Noe MH, Mehta NN, Gelfand JM. Psoriasis and the risk of diabetes: A prospective population-based cohort study. Journal of the American Academy of Dermatology. 2017. pii: S0190-9622(17)32616-6. DOI: 10.1016/j.jaad.2017.10.050. [Epub ahead of print]

[19] http://www.cancerresearchuk.org/about-us/cancerstats/faqs#How

[20] https://www.aihw.gov.au/reports/cancer/skin-cancer-in-australia/contents/ table-of-contents

[21] Miller JG, Neil SM. Gender and cutaneous melanoma. The British Journal of Dermatology. 1997;**136**:657-665

[22] Rumke P, Kleeberg UR, Mackie RM, Lejeune FJ, Planting AS, Brocker EB, Bierhorst JF, Lentz MA. Tamoxifen as a single agent for advanced melanoma in postmenopausal women. A phase II study of the EORTC malignant melanoma cooperative group. Melanoma Research. 1992;**2**:153-156

[23] Duncan LM, Travers RI, Koerner FC, Mihm MC Jr, Sober AJ. Estrogen and progesterone receptor analysis in pregnancy-associated melanoma: Absence of immunohistochemically detectable hormone receptors. Human Pathology. 1994;**25**:36-41

[24] Moroni G, Gaziano R, Bue C, Agostini M, Perno CF, Sinibaldi-Vallebona P, Pica F. Progesterone and melanoma cells: An old story suspended between life and death. Journal of Steroids Hormonal Science. 2015;**S13**:158. DOI: 10.4172/2157-7536.1000158

[25] Kanda N, Watanbe S. 17-β-estradiol, progesterone and dihydrotestosterone suppress the growth of human melanoma by inhibiting Interleukin-8 production. The Journal of Investigative Dermatology. 2001;**117**:274-283

[26] Reintgen DS, McCarty KS, Vollmer R, Cox E, Seigler HF. Malignant melanoma and pregnancy. Cancer. 1985;**55**:1340-1344

[27] McManamny DS, Moss ALH, Briggs JC, Pocock PV. Melanoma and pregnancy: A long-term follow-up. British Journal of Obstetrics and Gynaecology. 1989;**96**:1419-1423

[28] Mackie RM, Bufalino R, Morabito A, Cascinelli N, Sutherland C, Kroon BR, Urist M, Lejeune F, Hunter JA, Gohl J, Santi L, et al. Lack of effect of pregnancy on outcome of melanoma. Lancet. 1991;**337**:653-655

[29] Holly EA, Weiss NS, Liff JM. Cutaneous melanoma in relation to exogenous hormones and reproductive factors. Journal of the National Cancer Institute. 1983;**70**:827-831

[30] Stevens RG, Lee JAH, Moolgavkar SH. No association between oral contraceptives and malignant melanomas. The New England Journal of Medicine. 1980;**302**:966

[31] Green A, Bain C. Hormonal factors and melanoma in women. The Medical Journal of Australia. 1985;**142**:446-448

[32] Holman CDJ, Armstrong BK, Heenan PJ. Cutaneous malignant melanoma in women: Exogenous sex hormones and reproductive factors. British Journal of Cancer. 1984; **50**:673-680

[33] Ladanyi A, Timar J, Bocsi J, Towari J, Lapis K. Sex-dependent liver metastasis of human melanoma lines in SCID mice. Melanoma Research. 1995;**5**:83-86

[34] Feucht KA, Walker MJ, Das Gupta TK, Beattie CW. Effect of 17-β-oestradiol on the growth of estrogen receptor positive human melanoma in vitro and in athymic mice. Cancer Research. 1988;**48**:7093-7101

[35] Morvillo V, Luthy IA, Bravo AI, Capurro MI, Donaldson M, Quintans C, Calandra RS, Mordoh J. Atypical androgen receptor in the human melanoma cell line IIB-MEL-J. Pigment Cell Research. 1995;8(3):135-141

[36] Simanainen U, Ryan T, Li D, Suarez FG, Gao YR, Watson G, Wang Y, Handelsman DJ. Androgen receptor actions modify skin structure and chemical carcinogen-induced skin cancer susceptibility in mice. Hormones and Cancer. 2015;6:45-53

[37] Thomas-Ahner JM, Wulff BC, Tober KL, Kusewitt DF, Riggenbach JA, Oberyszyn TM. Gender differences in UV-B induced skin carcinogenesis, inflammation and DNA damage. Cancer Research. 2007;67(7):3468-3474. DOI: 10.1158/0008-5472.CAN-06-3798

[38] Zhu Y, Xiao Y, Wang J, Wan L, Yu T, Ma J, Liu J, Yu S, Jia L. Effects of metapristone and mifepristone (RU-486) on murine B16-F10 melanoma cancer metastasis abstracts. aaps. org/Verify/AAPS2014/PosterSubmissions/T3017.pdf

[39] Ghosh R, Ott AM, Seetharam D, Slaga TJ, Kumar AP. Cell cycle block and apoptosis induction in a human melanoma cell line following treatment with 2-methoxyostradiol: Therapeutic implications? Melanoma Research. 2003;13(2):119-127

[40] Lipkin G. Sex factors in growth of malignant melanoma in hamsters: In vivo and in vitro correlation. Cancer Research. 1970;30:1928-1930

[41] Disorbo DM, McNulty B, Nathanson L. In vitro growth inhibition of human malignant melanoma cells by glucocorticoids. Cancer Research. 1983;43:2664-2667

[42] De Luca M, Siegrist W, Bondanza S, Mathor M, Cancedda R, Eberle AN. α-Melanocyte stimulating hormone (α-MSH) stimulates normal human melanocyte growth by binding to high-affinity receptors. Journal of Cell Science. 1993;105:1079-1084

[43] Cos S, Garcia-Bolado A, Sanchez-Barcelo E. Direct antiproliferative effects of melatonin on two metastatic cell sub-lines of mouse melanoma (B16BL6 and PG19). Melanoma Research. 2001;11(2):197-201

[44] Ramaraj P, Cox JL. In-vitro effect of sex steroids on mouse melanoma (B16F10) cell growth. Cell Biology. 2014;3:60-71. http://dx.doi.org/10.4236/cellbio.2014.32007

[45] Ramaraj P, Cox JL. In-vitro effect of progesterone on human melanoma (BLM) cell growth. International Journal of Clinical and Experimental Medicine. 2014;7(11):3941-3953. PMID: 25550902: PMCID: PMC4276160

[46] Ramaraj P. In-vitro inhibition of human melanoma (BLM) cell growth by progesterone receptor antagonist RU-486 (Mifepristone). JCT. 2016;7(13):1045-1058. DOI: 10.4236/jct.2016.713101

[47] Seglen PO, Gordon PB. 3-Methyladenine: Specific inhibitior of autophagic/lysosomal protein degradation in isolated rat hepatocytes. Proceedings of the National Academy of Sciences. 1982;79:1889-1892

[48] Jagannath C, Lindsey DR, Dhandayuthapani S, Xu Y, Hunter RL Jr, Eissa NT. Autophagy enhances the efficacy of BCG vaccine by increasing peptide presentation in mouse dendritic cells. Nature Medicine. 2009;15(3):267-276

[49] Vegliante R, Desideri E, Di Leo L, Ciriolo R. Dehydroepiandrosterone triggers autophagic cell death in human hepatoma cell line HepG2 via JNK-mediated p62/SQSTM1 expression. Carcinogenesis. 2016;**37**(3):233-244

[50] Leder DC, Brown JR, Ramaraj P. In-vitro rescue and recovery studies of human melanoma (BLM) cell growth, adhesion and migration functions after treatment with progesterone. International Journal of Clinical and Experimental Medicine. 2015;**8**(8):12275-12285. PMID: 26550137 [PubMed] PMCID:PMC4612822

[51] Fang X, Zhang X, Zhou M, Li J. Effects of progesterone on the growth regulation in classical progesterone receptor-negative malignant melanoma cells. Journal of Huazhong University of Science and Technology Medical Sciences. 2010;**30**(2):231-234. DOI: 10.1007/s 11596-010-0220-3

Prognosis and Diagnosis Factors Studies

Chapter 4

CBX4 Expression and AFB1-Related Liver Cancer Prognosis

Qun-Ying Su, Jun Lu, Xiao-Ying Huang,
Jin-Guang Yao, Xue-Min Wu, Bing-Chen Huang,
Chao Wang, Qiang Xia and Xi-Dai Long

Additional information is available at the end of the chapter

http://dx.doi.org/10.5772/intechopen.78580

Abstract

Background: Previous studies have shown that chromobox 4 (CBX4) expression may involve in the progression of liver cancer, however, it is unclear whether it affects the prognosis of hepatocellular carcinoma (HCC) related to aflatoxin B1 (AFB1).

Methods: A retrospective study was conducted in the high AFB1 exposure areas and a total of 428 patients with HCC were included in the final survival analyses. AFB1 exposure levels and CBX4 expression in the tumor tissues were tested using enzyme-linked immunosorbent assay and immunohistochemistry, respectively. The effects of AFB1 and CBX4 on HCC outcome were elucidated by Kaplan–Meier survival method and Cox regression model.

Results: We found that the levels of AFB1 exposure and CBX4 expression in tumor tissues were significantly associated with some clinicopathological features such as microvessel density and tumor stage. Furthermore, both AFB1 and CBX4 significantly modified overall survival and tumor reoccurrence-free survival status of HCC. Additionally, some evidence of CBX4-AFB1 interaction affecting HCC prognosis was observed, with an interactive value of 1.98 for overall survival and 1.94 for tumor reoccurrence-free survival, respectively.

Conclusion: These results suggest that CBX4 expression might be a useful marker for AFB1-related HCC prognosis.

Keywords: CBX4, AFB1, HCC, prognosis

1. Introduction

Aflatoxin B1 (AFB1) is a type of secondary metabolite of *Aspergillus parasiticus* and *Aspergillus flavus*, and frequently contaminates a series of staple foods, such as ground nuts, and maize [1–3]. Once this type foods contaminated by AFB1 entered into human bodies, it is metabolized into its epoxides consisting of AFB1–8,9-exo-epoxide (AFBEX) and AFB1–8,9-endo-epoxide (AFBEN) by cytochrome P450 (CYP) metabolic system [3]. These products of AFB1, especially AFBEX, are characterized by high reaction, genic toxicity, and carcinogenicity [3]. Evidence from molecular epidemiology and animal models has shown that AFB1 is an important carcinogen inducing hepatocellular carcinoma (HCC) [4–10]. Mechanically, the carcinogenesis of AFB1-related HCC mainly involves in the formation of DNA damage (including AFB1-DNA adducts, DNA single-strand breaks, DNA double-strands breaks, and gene mutations), the inactivation of such tumor suppressor gene as TP53, and the activation of cancer genes such as Ras [3, 11–15]. Although some advance in the pathogenesis of AFB1-related HCC has obtained in the past decades [16–18], it is still far for us to elucidate more detailed mechanisms.

The chromobox 4 (Cbx4) (GenBank accession NO. 8535) consists of six exons and spans about 6.26 kb on chromosome 17q25.3. This gene encodes a 560-amino acid protein which is the important component of polycomb repressive complex 1 (PRC1) [19–22]. Functionally, CBX4 involves in PRC1-regulated transcription repression and post-translation modification [19–22]. Recently, increasing evidence has exhibited that the dysregulation of this gene may affect the carcinogenic process of some tumors such as HCC, colorectal cancer, breast cancer, and so on, and may be a significant prognostic biomarker [19, 21, 23–29]. However, it is not clear whether CBX4 modify the prognosis of AFB1-related HCC. Here, we conducted a hospital-based retrospective study to investigate whether the CBX4 expression in the cancerous tissues is associated with the outcome of HCC related to AFB1 expression in the Guangxi Region, a high AFB1 exposure area.

2. Materials and methods

2.1. Study population

Between January 2009 and December 2012, 428 consecutive patients with histopathologically confirmed hepatocarcinoma were recruited at the Divisions of Oncology and Pathology, the affiliated Hospitals of Guangxi Medical University and Youjiang Medical University for Nationalities. During the recruitment phase, only 5 cases refused to participate in the study (response rate 98.8%). All cases were from high AFB1 exposure areas, including Nanning, Bose, Tiandong, and Tianyang. After informed consent was obtained, surgically removed tumor samples were collected to analyze the amounts of AFB1-DNA adducts and CBX4 protein in the cancerous tissues. Additionally, all corresponding clinicopathological and survival following-up data were also collected in the hospitals as previously described methods [30-32]. In this study, the status of hepatitis B virus (HBV) and hepatitis C virus (HCV) infection was evaluated using serum hepatitis B surface antigen (HBsAg) and anti-HCV, respectively; whereas the grade and stage of tumor was elucidated using the Edmondson and Steiner (ES) grading system and the Barcelona Clinic Liver Cancer (BCLC) staging system, respectively. For survival analyses, the last follow-up day was set on December 31, 2017. The study protocol was carried out according to the approved guidelines by the Institutional Ethics Committee from the Affiliated Hospitals of Youjiang Medical University for Nationalities and Guangxi Medical University.

2.2. Microvessel density (MVD) assay

MVD in the cancerous tissues was assessed using the immunohistochemistry staining of CD31 as our previously described [30]. In this study, positive status of MVD was defined as microvessel counts more than 50 per ×200 magnifications.

2.3. AFB1 exposure data

AFB1 exposure levels were evaluated using the amounts of AFB1-DNA adducts in the cancerous tissues as our previously described [31, 32]. The amounts of AFB1-DNA adduct were tested using the competitive enzyme-linked immunosorbent assay. In this study, a value than less 1.00 μmol/mol DNA was considered as negative status for AFB1 exposure.

2.4. CBX4 expression assays

The level of CBX4 protein expression in cancerous tissues was elucidated using our previously published immunohistochemistry method [33, 34]. Briefly, the amounts of CBX4 protein were tested using anti-CBX4 antibody and calculated using immunoreactive score system (IRS). In the present study, positive CBX4 protein in cancerous tissues was define as IRS > 4.

2.5. Statistical analysis

Logistic regression model with enter method for variables (including all known clinicopathological features) was used for statistical comparison between groups. The odd ratios (ODs) and corresponding 95% confidence intervals (CIs) were calculated in this model for evaluating the association between clinicopathological features of HCCs and either AFB1 exposure or CBX4 expression. Kaplan–Meier survival method with log-rank test was used for statistical comparisons between different levels of AFB1 expression and CBX4 expression. Multivariate Cox regression model (with retread method based on likelihood ratio test) analyses were performed to calculate the risk strength of independent variates and prognostic values. In this study, all analyses were finished using the SPSS soft version 18.0 (SPSS Inc. Chicago, IL), and a P-value less than 0.05 was defined as statistical significance.

3. Results

3.1. The clinicopathological and survival features of HCC cases

Table 1 gave the clinicopathological characteristics of all cases, and a total of 428 patients with HCC were included in the final analyses. All cases were followed-up more than 5 years to obtain median survival time. During the follow-up period, 261 patients with

Variables	n	%
Total	428	100.0
Age, years		
Mean ± SE	47.9 ± 10.1	—
Range	30–75	—
Sex		
Man	290	68.9
Female	138	32.8
Ethnicity		
Han	229	54.4
Zhuang	199	47.3
HBV status		
HBsAg (−)	113	26.8
HBsAg (+)	315	74.8
HCV status		
anti-HCV (−)	378	89.8
anti-HCV (+)	50	11.9
Smoking status		
No	315	74.8
Yes	113	26.8
Drinking status		
No	304	72.2
Yes	124	29.5
AFP (ng/mL)		
≤ 20	154	36.6
> 20	274	65.1
Liver cirrhosis		
No	104	24.7
Yes	324	77.0
BCLC stage		
A	167	39.7
B	121	28.7
C	140	33.3
Tumor size		
≤ 3 cm	211	50.1
> 3 cm	217	51.5
MVD		
Negative	192	45.6

Variables	n	%
Positive	236	56.1
ES grade		
Low	226	53.7
High	202	48.0

Abbreviations: AFP, α-fetoprotein; BCLC, the Barcelona Clinic Liver Cancer staging system; ES, Edmondson and Steiner grading system; HBsAg, hepatitis B surface antigen; HBV, hepatitis B virus; HCV, hepatitis C virus; MVD, microvessel density.

Table 1. The clinic-pathological features of cases with hepatocellular carcinoma.

HCC featured cancer recurrences with 30.00 (22.20–37.80) months of median recurrence-free survival time (MRT), and 270 died with 45.00 (38.98–51.02) months of median overall survival time (MST).

3.2. The effects of AFB1 exposure on the clinicopathological features and the prognosis of HCC cases

In this study, the status of AFB1 exposure was elucidated using the amount of AFB1-DNA adducts in the cancerous tissues. Results from competitive ELISA exhibited the patients with HCC featured a 2.82 ± 1.60 μmol/mol DNA of AFB1 exposure level. To investigate the effects of AFB1 exposure on the clinicopathological features of HCC cases, we defined the amount of AFB1-DNA adducts ≤1.00 μmol/mol DNA as negative AFB1 exposure according to our previous published results [31, 32]. Our results showed that these patients with positive AFB1 status (AFB1-DNA adducts: > 1.00 μmol/mol DNA) had higher BCLC stage (adjusted OR = 2.09 and adjusted 95% CI = 1.04–4.24), bigger tumor size (adjusted OR = 69.06 and adjusted 95% CI = 33.62–141.86), and higher MVD (adjusted OR = 2.56 and adjusted 95% CI = 1.36–4.81) compared with those without positive AFB1 status (OR = 1) (**Table 2**). Additionally, we also found that the levels of AFB1 exposure were significantly associated with the age of patients with hepatocarcinoma (adjusted OR = 1.80, adjusted 95% CI = 1.22–2.66, and $P = 3.07 \times 10^{-3}$). However, AFB1 exposure was not correlated with other clinicopathological features of HCCs (**Table 2**).

Next, we investigated the effects of AFB1 exposure on the HCC prognosis using Kaplan–Meier survival model (**Figure 1A**). Results exhibited that HCC cases with negative AFB1 status (AFB1-DNA adducts: ≤ 1.00 μmol/mol DNA) featured longer median overall survival time (MST) [69.00 (55.41–82.59) months] and median tumor reoccurrence-free survival time (MRT) [70.00 (44.93–95.07) months] compared with those with positive AFB1 status [20.00 (13.04–26.96) months for MST and 13.00 (9.54–16.46) months for MRT, respectively].

3.3. The effects of CBX4 expression on the clinicopathological features and the prognosis of HCC cases

In the present, the levels of CBX4 protein in the cancerous tissues were amounted using immunohistochemistry technique with IRS counting system and the median IRS value was 5.58 for

Variables	AFB1 (−)		AFB1 (+)		OR (95% CI)	P_{trend}
	n	%	n	%		
Total	244	100.0	184	100.0	—	—
Age (years)						
≤ 48	148	60.7	86	46.7	Reference	
> 48	96	39.3	98	53.3	1.80 (1.22–2.66)	3.07×10^{-3}
Sex						
Man	160	65.6	130	70.7	Reference	
Female	84	34.4	54	29.3	1.13 (0.59–2.13)	0.72
Ethnicity						
Han	124	50.8	105	57.1	Reference	
Zhuang	120	49.2	79	42.9	0.99 (0.55–1.78)	0.98
HBsAg						
Negative	65	26.6	48	26.1	Reference	
Positive	179	73.4	136	73.9	1.19 (0.60–2.34)	0.61
anti-HCV						
Negative	217	88.9	161	87.5	Reference	
Positive	27	11.1	23	12.5	1.25 (0.51–3.09)	0.62
Smoking status						
No	181	74.2	134	72.8	Reference	
Yes	63	25.8	50	27.2	0.48 (0.12–1.85)	0.28
Drinking status						
No	174	71.3	130	70.7	Reference	
Yes	70	28.7	54	29.3	2.61 (0.69–9.89)	0.27
AFP (ng/mL)						
≤ 20	82	33.6	72	39.1	Reference	
> 20	162	66.4	112	60.9	1.00 (0.55–1.82)	0.99
Liver cirrhosis						
No	58	23.8	46	25.0	Reference	
Yes	186	76.2	138	75.0	0.84 (0.42–1.69)	0.63
BCLC stage						
A	113	46.3	54	29.3	Reference	
B	69	28.3	52	28.3	1.27 (0.61–2.61)	0.52
C	62	25.4	78	42.4	2.09 (1.04–4.24)	0.04
Tumor size						
≤ 3 cm	197	80.7	14	7.6	Reference	

Variables	AFB1 (–)		AFB1 (+)		OR (95% CI)	P_{trend}
	n	%	n	%		
> 3 cm	47	19.3	170	92.4	69.06 (33.62–141.86)	9.36×10^{-31}
MVD						
Negative	118	48.4	74	40.2	Reference	
Positive	126	51.6	110	59.8	2.56 (1.36–4.81)	3.46×10^{-3}
ES grade						
Low	129	52.9	97	52.7	Reference	
High	115	47.1	87	47.3	1.52 (0.64–2.07)	0.64

Abbreviations: AFP, α-fetoprotein; BCLC, the Barcelona Clinic Liver Cancer staging system; ES, Edmondson and Steiner grading system; HBsAg, hepatitis B surface antigen; HBV, hepatitis B virus; HCV, hepatitis C virus; MVD, microvessel density.

Table 2. The association between AFB1 exposure and clinic-pathological features of hepatocellular carcinoma cases.

all cases with hepatocarcinoma. According to the results from the CBX4 expression in cancerous tissues based on a large sample, IRS > 4 was regarded as positive CBX4 status. **Table 3** summarized the association between CBX4 expression in the cancerous tissues and the clinicopathological features, and results from multivariable logistic regression models proved that the levels of CBX4 expression were significantly related to increasing risk of liver cirrhosis (OR = 1.75 and 95% CI = 1.07–2.88), higher tumor stage (OR = 2.02 and 95% CI = 1.23–3.33), and increasing MVD (OR = 2.66 and 95% CI = 1.74–4.07). However, CBX4 expression levels did not affect other clinicopathological features such as tumor size, grade, AFP, and so on.

Results from Kaplan–Meier survival analyses further displayed that HCC patients with positive status of CBX4 protein expression had short MST [22.00 (18.00–26.00) months] and MRT [16.00 (10.88–21.12) months] compared with those with negative-status CBX4 protein [69.00 (52.75–85.25) months for MST and 48.00 (23.69–72.31) months for MRT, respectively] (**Figure 1B**). Taken together, CBX4 expression in the cancerous might be an important biomarker for HCC prognosis.

3.4. The joint effects of AFB1 exposure and CBX4 expression on HCC prognosis

Given that both AFB1 exposure and CBX4 expression modified HCC outcome, we questioned whether CBX4 expression interacted with AFB1 expression, and whether this interaction affected the prognosis of hepatocarcinoma. First, we analyzed the joint effects of AFB1 exposure and CBX4 expression on the prognosis of patients with HCC using Kaplan–Meier survival model (**Figure 2**). In this model, the combination of AFB1 exposure and CBX4 expression was divided into four groups: cases with negative-AFB1 and negative-CBX4 status (AC-1), cases with negative-AFB1 and positive-CBX4 status (AC-2), cases with positive-AFB1 and negative-CBX4 status (AC-3), and cases with positive-AFB1 and positive-CBX4 status (AC-4). We found MST and MRT gradually decreased from AC-1 to AC-4 (89.00–11.00 months for MST and more than 125.00–7.00 months for MRT, respectively) (**Figure 2A** and **B**).

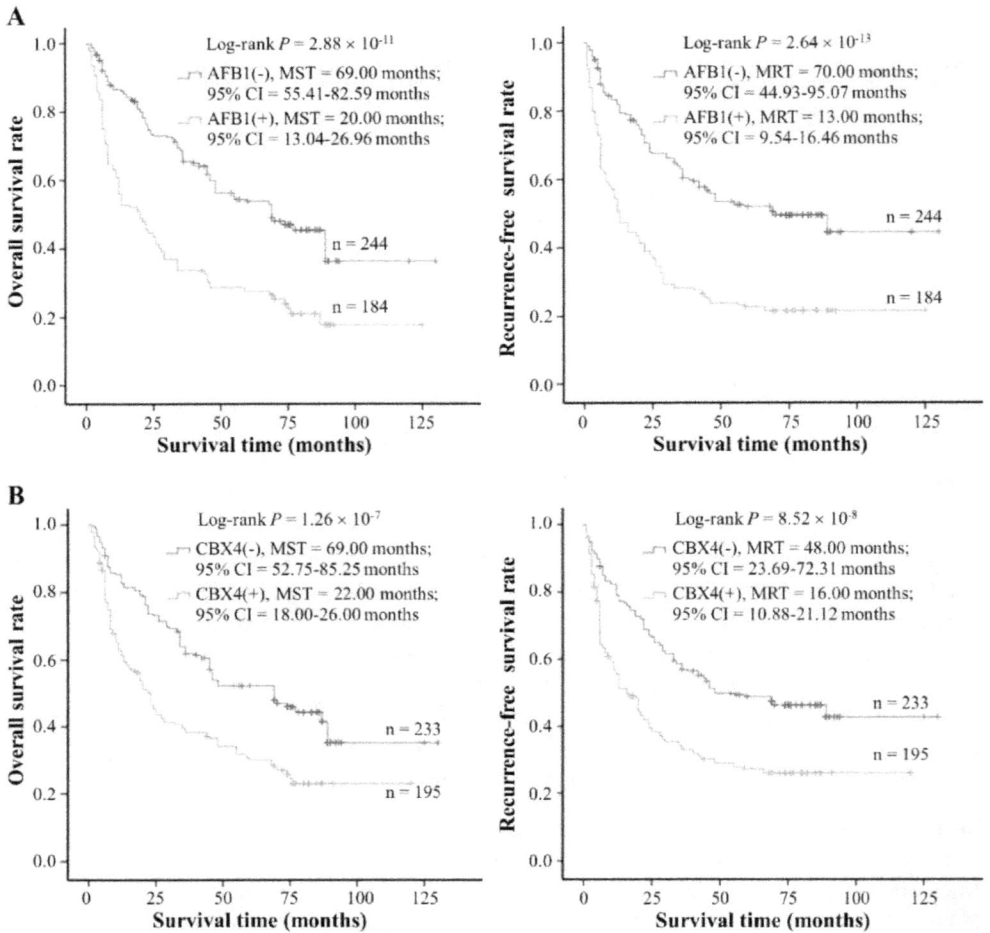

Figure 1. Both AFB1 exposure and CBX4 expression significantly correlating with hepatocellular carcinoma. AFB1 exposure levels were elucidated using the amount of AFB1-DNA adducts in the cancerous tissues. The CBX4 expression in cancerous tissues from 428 patients with hepatocellular carcinoma was tested using immunohistochemistry technique based on immunoreactive score system (IRS). To analyze, the levels of CBX4 expression were divided into two groups: Negative group (IRS ≤ 4) and positive group (IRS > 4). AFB1 exposure (A) and CBX4 expression (B) are associated with overall survival (left) and tumor recurrence-free survival (right) of hepatocellular carcinoma. Cumulative hazard function was plotted by Kaplan–Meier's methodology, and P value was calculated with two-sided log-rank tests. *Abbreviations:* CBX4, chromobox 4; MST, median overall survival time; MRT, median tumor recurrence-free survival time; CI, confidence interval.

We next finished multivariable Cox regression analyses based on the retread method with likelihood ratio test (including significant variables and all kinds of possible interactive variables) (**Table 4**), and found both AFB1 exposure and CBX4 expression in the cancerous tissues were independent prognostic factors. Furthermore, we also observed that AFB1 exposure significantly and multiplicatively interacted with CBX4 protein expression (interactive values, 1.98 for overall survival and 1.94 for tumor reoccurrence-free survival, respectively).

Variables	CBX4 (−)		CBX4 (+)		OR (95% CI)	P_{trend}
	n	%	n	%		
Total	233	100.0	195	100.0	—	—
Age (years)						
≤ 48	136	58.4	98	50.3	Reference	
> 48	97	41.6	97	49.7	1.35 (0.89–2.05)	0.67
Sex						
Man	160	68.7	130	66.7	Reference	
Female	73	31.3	65	33.3	1.14 (0.73–1.78)	0.57
Ethnicity						
Han	121	51.9	108	55.4	Reference	
Zhuang	112	48.1	87	44.6	0.96 (0.63–1.46)	0.85
HBsAg						
Negative	65	27.9	48	24.6	Reference	
Positive	168	72.1	148	75.9	1.17 (0.73–1.89)	0.51
anti-HCV						
Negative	209	89.7	169	86.7	Reference	
Positive	24	10.3	26	13.3	1.43 (0.74–2.75)	0.29
Smoking status						
No	176	75.5	139	71.3	Reference	
Yes	57	24.5	56	28.7	1.04 (0.37–2.93)	0.94
Drinking status						
No	172	73.8	132	67.7	Reference	
Yes	61	26.2	63	32.3	1.40 (0.51–3.83)	0.51
AFP (ng/mL)						
≤ 20	84	36.1	70	35.9	Reference	
> 20	149	63.9	125	64.1	1.11 (0.72–1.70)	0.64
Liver cirrhosis						
No	69	29.6	35	17.9	Reference	
Yes	164	70.4	160	82.1	1.75 (1.07–2.88)	0.03
BCLC stage						
A	112	48.1	55	28.2	Reference	
B	58	24.9	63	32.3	1.94 (1.16–3.24)	0.01
C	63	27.0	77	39.5	2.02 (1.23–3.33)	5.79×10^{-3}
Tumor size						
≤ 3 cm	121	51.9	90	46.2	Reference	
> 3 cm	112	48.1	105	53.8	1.24 (0.81–1.88)	0.33

	CBX4 (–)		CBX4 (+)			
MVD						
Negative	131	56.2	61	31.3	Reference	
Positive	102	43.8	134	68.7	2.66 (1.74–4.07)	6.65×10^{-6}
ES grade						
Low	132	56.7	94	48.2	Reference	
High	101	43.3	101	51.8	1.39 (0.92–2.11)	0.12

Abbreviations: AFP, α-fetoprotein; BCLC, the Barcelona Clinic Liver Cancer staging system; CBX4, chromobox 4; ES, Edmondson and Steiner grading system; HBsAg, hepatitis B surface antigen; HBV, hepatitis B virus; HCV, hepatitis C virus; MVD, microvessel density.

Table 3. The correlation between CBX4 expression and clinical pathological features of hepatocellular carcinoma.

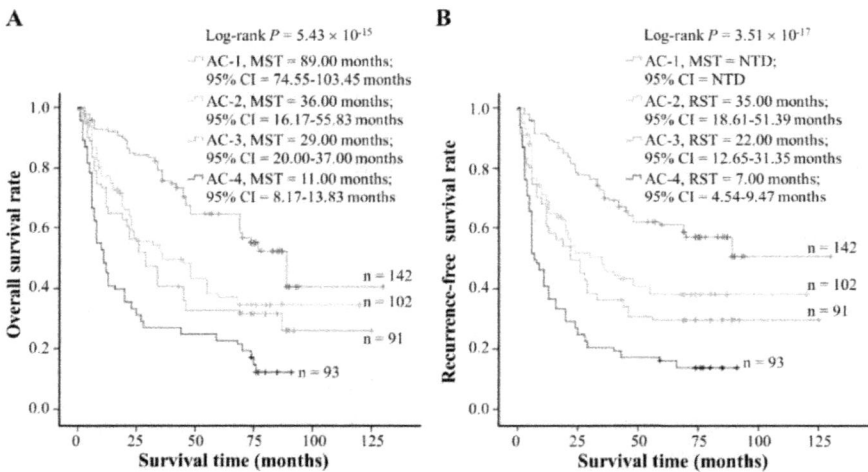

Figure 2. Survival analysis of CBX4 expression binding AFB1 exposure levels. The combination of CBX4 expression and AFB1 exposure was divided into 4 strata: Cases with negative-AFB1 and negative-CBX4 status (AC-1), cases with negative-AFB1 and positive-CBX4 status (AC-2), cases with positive-AFB1 and negative-CBX4 status (AC-3), and cases with positive-AFB1 and positive-CBX4 status (AC-4). This kind of joint analyses showed that interactive effects on the overall survival (A) and tumor recurrence-free survival (B) of patients with hepatocarcinoma. Cumulative hazard function was plotted by Kaplan–Meier's methodology, and *P* value was calculated with two-sided log-rank tests. *Abbreviations:* CBX4, chromobox 4; MST, median overall survival time; MRT, median tumor recurrence-free survival time; CI, confidence interval.

4. Discussion

In Guangxi Zhuang Autonomous Region, HCC is the most malignant disease. In the past decades, the annual incidence and death rate (AIR and ADR) of hepatocarcinoma in this area has been reported to remarkably increase (up to about 100–200 per 10,000 for AIR about 50 per 10,000 for ADR) [1]. Lots of epidemiological studies have shown that AFB1 exposure is

Variables	OS		RFS	
	HR (95%CI)	Ptrend	HR (95%CI)	Ptrend
AFB1	2.09 (1.64–2.65)	2.34×10^{-9}	2.29 (1.79–2.93)	3.82×10^{-11}
CBX4	1.76 (1.38–2.24)	4.66×10^{-6}	1.80 (1.41–2.30)	3.12×10^{-6}
AFB1 × CBX4	1.98 (1.61–2.59)	9.43×10^{-7}	1.94 (1.58–2.54)	8.17×10^{-5}

HR and corresponding 95% CI was calculated using multivariable Cox regression model (with retread method based on likelihood ratio test). *Abbreviations:* AFB1, aflatoxin B1; CBX4, chromobox 4; OS, overall survival; RFS, tumor reoccurrence-free survival; HR, hazard ratio; CI, confidence interval.

Table 4. The effects of AFB1 and CBX4 expression on the prognosis of cases with hepatocellular carcinoma.

the most important cause for this high AIR and ADR [1]. AFB1 is a known I-type chemical carcinogen produced by *Aspergillus parasiticus* and *Aspergillus flavus*, and has been proved to involve in the carcinogenesis and progression of HCC [4–10]. This carcinogenicity of AFB1 mainly results from its metabolic product binding to DNA and inducing DNA damage. Among DNA damage types induced by AFB1, AFB1-DNA adducts are very important, because of its non-enzymatic, time-dependent, and apparent persistent characteristics in the genomic DNA strands [3, 35]. Our previous studies have exhibited that AFB1-DNA adducts, especially from liver tissues, are highly associated not only with increasing HCC risk, but with the poor prognosis of HCC [2, 31, 36–39]. Here, our data displayed that increasing levels of AFB1 exposure significantly correlated with higher tumor stage, increasing tumor size, and higher MVD; furthermore, AFB1 was also poor prognostic marker for HCC. Taken together, these data suggest that AFB1 may involve in the startup and progression of HCC.

Because several previous studies have exhibited that CBX4 can progress tumorigenesis via several signal pathways, including CBX4/HIF-1α/VEGF pathway [20, 25, 26, 34], CBX4/HDAC3/Runx2 pathway [21], CBX4/P63 pathway [22], CBX4/miR-195 pathway [40], CBX4/CtIP pathway [41], and CBX4/P53 pathway [42, 43], here we investigated the effects of CXB4 expression on HCC outcome. We not only found that increasing CBX4 expression in the cancerous tissues is a poor prognostic biomarker for HCC, but this increasing expression is associated with clinicopathological features such as tumor size, tumor stage, and angiogenesis. Supporting our findings, several recent reports further prove that CBX4 can govern the several biofunctions of HCC, including proliferation, invasion and metastasis, angiogenesis, and metastasis [20, 25, 26, 34, 40, 44].

Noticeably, some evidence of the joint effects of CBX4 and AFB1 on HCC outcome was observed in the prognostic analyses based on the gene-environmental joint effects. Our results showed that CBX4 expression significantly and multiplicatively interacted with AFB1 exposure levels, and that this multiplicative interaction remarkably increased the death risk and tumor reoccurrence risk of patients with HCC. Recently, two studies from high AFB1 exposure areas have also reported that the dysregulation of CBX4 in the cancerous tissues from patients with hepatocarcinoma increases MVD, promotes angiogenesis, and increases sensitivity of HCC cells on anti-cancer drugs [33, 34]. Altogether, these results are indicative of the angiogenesis induced by CBX4 involving in the progression of AFB1-related HCC.

In summary, our present study proposes that CBX4 expression in the cancerous tissues can act as a valuable biomarker for AFB1-related HCC. However, several limitations confine the value of this study. First, because of the hospital-based retrospective design, selective bias may take place. Second, because liver damage itself affects AFB1 metabolite and may increase the amount of AFB1-DNA adducts, the prognostic and interactive values of AFB1 and CBX4 may be underestimated. Finally, we did not do functional and mechanical analyses. Therefore, detailed functional analyses deserve further evaluation on the basis of the foresighted design and the combination of AFB1 and CBX4.

Conflicts of interest and source of funding

The authors declare no competing financial interests. This study was supported in part by the National Natural Science Foundation of China (Nos. 81,760,502, 81,572,353, 81,372,639, 81,472,243, 81,660,495, and 81,460,423), the Innovation Program of Guangxi Municipal Education Department (Nos. 201204LX674 and 201204LX324), Innovation Program of Guangxi Health Department (No. Z2013781), the Natural Science Foundation of Guangxi (Nos. 2017GXNSFAA198002, 2017GXNSFGA198002, 2016GXNSFDA380003, 2015GXNSFAA139223, 2013GXNSFAA019251, 2014GXNSFDA118021, and 2014GXNSFAA118144), Research Program of Guangxi "Zhouyue Scholar" (No. 2017–2038), Research Program of Guangxi Specially invited Expert (No. 2017-6th), Research Program of Guangxi Clinic Research Center of Hepatobiliary Diseases (No.AD17129025), and Open Research Program from Molecular Immunity Study Room Involving in Acute & Severe Diseases in Guangxi Colleges and Universities (Nos. kfkt20160062 and kfkt20160063).

Abbreviations

AFB1	aflatoxin B1
AFBEX	AFB1–8,9-exo-epoxide
AFBEN	AFB1–8,9-endo-epoxide
BCLC	The Barcelona Clinic Liver Cancer
CBX4	chromobox 4
CI	confidence interval
CYP	cytochrome P450
ES	The Edmondson and Steiner
HBV	hepatitis B virus
HCC	hepatocellular carcinoma
HCV	hepatitis C virus

HBsAg   hepatitis B surface antigen

IRS   immunoreactive score system

MRT   median tumor reoccurrence-free survival time

MST   median overall survival time

MVD   microvessel density

OD   odd ratio.

Author details

Qun-Ying Su[1], Jun Lu[2], Xiao-Ying Huang[1], Jin-Guang Yao[1], Xue-Min Wu[1],
Bing-Chen Huang[1], Chao Wang[3], Qiang Xia[2] and Xi-Dai Long[1,2,4*]

*Address all correspondence to: sjtulongxd@263.net

1 Department of Pathology, The Affiliated Hospital of Youjiang Medical University for
Nationalities, Baise, China

2 Department of Liver Surgery, Renji Hospital, School of Medicine, Shanghai Jiao Tong
University, Shanghai, China

3 Department of Digestive Medicine, The Affiliated Hospital of Youjiang Medical University
for Nationalities, Baise, China

4 Guangxi Clinic Research Center of Hepatobiliary Diseases, Baise, China

References

[1] Wu XM, Xi ZF, Lu J, Wang XZ, Zhang TQ, Huang XY, Yao JG, Wang C, Wei ZH, Luo CY,
Huang BC, Xu QQ, Yang WP, Xia Q, Long XD. Genetic single nucleotide polymorphisms
(GSNPs) in the DNA repair genes and hepatocellular carcinoma related to aflatoxin B1
among Guangxiese population. In: Parine NR, editor. Genetic Polymorphisms. Vol. 1.
Rijeka, Croatia: InTech; 2017. pp. 97-119. DOI: 10.5772/intechopen.69530

[2] Long XD, Yao JD, Yang Q, Huang CH, Liao P, Nong LG, Tang YJ, Huang XY, Wang C,
Wu XM, Huang BC, Ban FZ, Zeng LX, Ma Y, Zhai B, Zhang JQ, Xue F, Lu CX, Xia Q.
Polymorphisms of DNA repair genes and toxicological effects of aflatoxin B1 exposure.
In: Faulkner AG, editor. Aflatoxins: Food Sources, Occurrence and Toxicological Effects.
1st ed. New York: Nova Science Publishers; 2014. pp. 125-156. DOI: 978-1-63117-298-4

[3] Kew MC. Aflatoxins as a cause of hepatocellular carcinoma. Journal of Gastrointestinal
and Liver Diseases. 2013;**22**:305-310

[4] Rushing BR, Selim MI. Adduction to arginine detoxifies aflatoxin B1 by eliminating genotoxicity and altering in vitro toxicokinetic profiles. Oncotarget. 2018;9:4559-4570. DOI: 10.18632/oncotarget.23382

[5] Xiang X, Qin HG, You XM, Wang YY, Qi LN, Ma L, Xiang BD, Zhong JH, Li LQ. Expression of P62 in hepatocellular carcinoma involving hepatitis B virus infection and aflatoxin B1 exposure. Cancer Medicine. 2017;6:2357-2369. DOI: 10.1002/cam4.1176

[6] Weng MW, Lee HW, Choi B, Wang HT, Hu Y, Mehta M, Desai D, Amin S, Zheng Y, Tang MS. AFB1 hepatocarcinogenesis is via lipid peroxidation that inhibits DNA repair, sensitizes mutation susceptibility and induces aldehyde-DNA adducts at p53 mutational hotspot codon 249. Oncotarget. 2017;8:18213-18226. DOI: 10.18632/oncotarget.15313

[7] Narkwa PW, Blackbourn DJ, Mutocheluh M. Aflatoxin B1 inhibits the type 1 interferon response pathway via STAT1 suggesting another mechanism of hepatocellular carcinoma. Infectious Agents and Cancer. 2017;12:17. DOI: 10.1186/s13027-017-0127-8

[8] Maurya BK, Trigun SK. Fisetin attenuates AKT associated growth promoting events in AflatoxinB1 induced hepatocellular carcinoma. Anti-Cancer Agents in Medicinal Chemistry. 2017. DOI: 10.2174/1871520618666171229223335. E-pub Ahead of Print

[9] Huang MN, Yu W, Teoh WW, Ardin M, Jusakul A, Ng AWT, Boot A, Abedi-Ardekani B, Villar S, Myint SS, Othman R, Poon SL, Heguy A, Olivier M, Hollstein M, Tan P, Teh BT, Sabapathy K, Zavadil J, Rozen SG. Genome-scale mutational signatures of aflatoxin in cells, mice, and human tumors. Genome Research. 2017;27:1475-1486. DOI: 10.1101/gr.220038.116

[10] Chu YJ, Yang HI, Wu HC, Liu J, Wang LY, Lu SN, Lee MH, Jen CL, You SL, Santella RM, Chen CJ. Aflatoxin B1 exposure increases the risk of cirrhosis and hepatocellular carcinoma in chronic hepatitis B virus carriers. International Journal of Cancer. 2017;141:711-720. DOI: 10.1002/ijc.30782

[11] Chawanthayatham S, Valentine CC, 3rd, Fedeles BI, Fox EJ, Loeb LA, Levine SS, Slocum SL, Wogan GN, Croy RG, Essigmann JM. Mutational spectra of aflatoxin B1 in vivo establish biomarkers of exposure for human hepatocellular carcinoma. Proceedings of the National Academy of Sciences of the United States of America. 2017;114:E3101-E3109. DOI: 10.1073/pnas.1700759114

[12] Umesha S, Manukumar HM, Chandrasekhar B, Shivakumara P, Shiva Kumar J, Raghava S, Avinash P, Shirin M, Bharathi TR, Rajini SB, Nandhini M, Vinaya Rani GG, Shobha M, Prakash HS. Aflatoxins and food pathogens: Impact of biologically active aflatoxins and their control strategies. Journal of the Science of Food and Agriculture. 2017;97:1698-1707. DOI: 10.1002/jsfa.8144

[13] Sarma UP, Bhetaria PJ, Devi P, Varma A. Aflatoxins: Implications on health. Indian Journal of Clinical Biochemistry. 2017;32:124-133. DOI: 10.1007/s12291-017-0649-2

[14] Kowalska A, Walkiewicz K, Koziel P, Muc-Wierzgon M. Aflatoxins: Characteristics and impact on human health. Postępy Higieny i Medycyny Doświadczalnej (Online). 2017;71:315-327. DOI: 10.5604/01.3001.0010.3816

[15] Woloshuk CP, Shim WB. Aflatoxins, fumonisins, and trichothecenes: A convergence of knowledge. FEMS Microbiology Reviews. 2013;**37**:94-109. DOI: 10.1111/1574-6976.12009

[16] Khlangwiset P, Shephard GS, Wu F. Aflatoxins and growth impairment: A review. Critical Reviews in Toxicology. 2011;**41**:740-755. DOI: 10.3109/10408444.2011.575766

[17] Wu Q, Jezkova A, Yuan Z, Pavlikova L, Dohnal V, Kuca K. Biological degradation of aflatoxins. Drug Metabolism Reviews. 2009;**41**:1-7. DOI: 10.1080/03602530802563850

[18] Villar S, Ortiz-Cuaran S, Abedi-Ardekani B, Gouas D, Nogueira da Costa A, Plymoth A, Khuhaprema T, Kalalak A, Sangrajrang S, Friesen MD, Groopman JD, Hainaut P. Aflatoxin-induced TP53 R249S mutation in hepatocellular carcinoma in Thailand: Association with tumors developing in the absence of liver cirrhosis. PLoS One. 2012; **7**:e37707. DOI: 10.1371/journal.pone.0037707

[19] Zeng JS, Zhang ZD, Pei L, Bai ZZ, Yang Y, Yang H, Tian QH. CBX4 exhibits oncogenic activities in breast cancer via Notch1 signaling. The International Journal of Biochemistry & Cell Biology. 2018;**95**:1-8. DOI: 10.1016/j.biocel.2017.12.006

[20] Yang J, Cheng D, Zhu B, Zhou S, Ying T, Yang Q. Chromobox homolog 4 is positively correlated to tumor growth, survival and activation of HIF-1alpha signaling in human osteosarcoma under normoxic condition. Journal of Cancer. 2016;**7**:427-435. DOI: 10.7150/jca.13749

[21] Wang X, Li L, Wu Y, Zhang R, Zhang M, Liao D, Wang G, Qin G, Xu RH, Kang T. CBX4 suppresses metastasis via recruitment of HDAC3 to the Runx2 promoter in colorectal carcinoma. Cancer Research. 2016;**76**:7277-7289. DOI: 10.1158/0008-5472.CAN-16-2100

[22] Cohen I, Ezhkova E. Cbx4: A new guardian of p63's domain of epidermal control. The Journal of Cell Biology. 2016;**212**:9-11. DOI: 10.1083/jcb.201512032

[23] Liang YK, Lin HY, Chen CF, Zeng. Prognostic values of distinct CBX family members in breast cancer. Oncotarget. 2017;**8**:92375-92387. DOI: 10.18632/oncotarget.21325

[24] Lin FM, Kumar S, Ren J, Karami S, Bahnassy S, Li Y, Zheng X, Wang J, Bawa-Khalfe T. SUMOylation of HP1alpha supports association with ncRNA to define responsiveness of breast cancer cells to chemotherapy. Oncotarget. 2016;**7**:30336-30349. DOI: 10.18632/oncotarget.8733

[25] Mei Z, Jiao H, Wang W, Li J, Chen G, Xu Y. Polycomb chromobox 4 enhances migration and pulmonary metastasis of hepatocellular carcinoma cell line MHCC97L. Science China. Life Sciences. 2014;**57**:610-617. DOI: 10.1007/s11427-014-4663-9

[26] Li J, Xu Y, Jiao H, Wang W, Mei Z, Chen G. Sumoylation of hypoxia inducible factor-1alpha and its significance in cancer. Science China. Life Sciences. 2014;**57**:657-664. DOI: 10.1007/s11427-014-4685-3

[27] Oh Y, Chung KC. Small ubiquitin-like modifier (SUMO) modification of zinc finger protein 131 potentiates its negative effect on estrogen signaling. The Journal of Biological Chemistry. 2012;**287**:17517-17529. DOI: 10.1074/jbc.M111.336354

[28] Ismail IH, Gagne JP, Caron MC, McDonald D, Xu Z, Masson JY, Poirier GG, Hendzel MJ. CBX4-mediated SUMO modification regulates BMI1 recruitment at sites of DNA damage. Nucleic Acids Research. 2012;**40**:5497-5510. DOI: 10.1093/nar/gks222

[29] Vandamme J, Volkel P, Rosnoblet C, Le Faou P, Angrand PO. Interaction proteomics analysis of polycomb proteins defines distinct PRC1 complexes in mammalian cells. Molecular & Cellular Proteomics. 2011;**10**:M110-M002642. DOI: 10.1074/mcp.M110.002642

[30] Liu YX, Long XD, Xi ZF, Ma Y, Huang XY, Yao JG, Wang C, Xing TY, Xia Q. MicroRNA-24 modulates aflatoxin B1-related hepatocellular carcinoma prognosis and tumorigenesis. BioMed Research International. 2014;**2014**:482926. DOI: 10.1155/2014/482926

[31] Long XD, Yao JG, Zeng Z, Ma Y, Huang XY, Wei ZH, Liu M, Zhang JJ, Xue F, Zhai B, Xia Q. Polymorphisms in the coding region of X-ray repair complementing group 4 and aflatoxin B1-related hepatocellular carcinoma. Hepatology. 2013;**58**:171-181. DOI: 10.1002/hep.26311

[32] Long XD, Ma Y, Huang HD, Yao JG, Qu de Y, Lu YL. Polymorphism of XRCC1 and the frequency of mutation in codon 249 of the p53 gene in hepatocellular carcinoma among Guangxi population, china. Molecular Carcinogenesis. 2008;**47**:295-300. DOI: 10.1002/mc.20384

[33] Jiao HK, Xu Y, Li J, Wang W, Mei Z, Long XD, Chen GQ. Prognostic significance of Cbx4 expression and its beneficial effect for transarterial chemoembolization in hepatocellular carcinoma. Cell Death & Disease. 2015;**6**:e1689. DOI: 10.1038/cddis.2015.57

[34] Li J, Xu Y, Long XD, Wang W, Jiao HK, Mei Z, Yin QQ, Ma LN, Zhou AW, Wang LS, Yao M, Xia Q, Chen GQ. Cbx4 governs HIF-1alpha to potentiate angiogenesis of hepatocellular carcinoma by its SUMO E3 ligase activity. Cancer Cell. 2014;**25**:118-131. DOI: 10.1016/j.ccr.2013.12.008

[35] Kensler TW, Roebuck BD, Wogan GN, Groopman JD. Aflatoxin: A 50-year odyssey of mechanistic and translational toxicology. Toxicological Sciences. 2011;**120**(Suppl 1):S28-S48. DOI: 10.1093/toxsci/kfq283

[36] Yao JG, Huang XY, Long XD. Interaction of DNA repair gene polymorphisms and aflatoxin B1 in the risk of hepatocellular carcinoma. International Journal of Clinical and Experimental Pathology. 2014;**7**:6231-6244. DOI: 10.2016/1936-2625.25337275

[37] Long XD, Zhao D, Wang C, Huang XY, Yao JG, Ma Y, Wei ZH, Liu M, Zeng LX, Mo XQ, Zhang JJ, Xue F, Zhai B, Xia Q. Genetic polymorphisms in DNA repair genes XRCC4 and XRCC5 and aflatoxin B1-related hepatocellular carcinoma. Epidemiology. 2013;**24**:671-681. DOI: 10.1097/EDE.0b013e31829d2744

[38] Long XD, Yao JG, Zeng Z, Huang CH, Huang ZS, Huang YZ, Ban FZ, Huang XY, Yao LM, Fan LD, Fu GH. DNA repair capacity-related to genetic polymorphisms of DNA repair genes and aflatoxin B1-related hepatocellular carcinoma among Chinese population. In: Kruman I, editor. DNA Repair. Rijeka, Croatia: InTech; 2011. pp. 505-524. DOI: 10.5772/20792

[39] Long XD, Ma Y, Zhou YF, Ma AM, Fu GH. Polymorphism in xeroderma pigmentosum complementation group C codon 939 and aflatoxin B1-related hepatocellular carcinoma in the Guangxi population. Hepatology. 2010;**52**:1301-1309. DOI: 10.1002/hep.23807

[40] Zheng C, Li J, Wang Q, Liu W, Zhou J, Liu R, Zeng Q, Peng X, Huang C, Cao P, Cao K. microRNA-195 functions as a tumor suppressor by inhibiting CBX4 in hepatocellular carcinoma. Oncology Reports. 2015;**33**:1115-1122. DOI: 10.3892/or.2015.3734

[41] Soria-Bretones I, Cepeda-Garcia C, Checa-Rodriguez C, Heyer V, Reina-San-Martin B, Soutoglou E, Huertas P. DNA end resection requires constitutive sumoylation of CtIP by CBX4. Nature Communications. 2017;**8**:113. DOI: 10.1038/s41467-017-00183-6

[42] Peuget S, Bonacci T, Soubeyran P, Iovanna J, Dusetti NJ. Oxidative stress-induced p53 activity is enhanced by a redox-sensitive TP53INP1 SUMOylation. Cell Death and Differentiation. 2014;**21**:1107-1118. DOI: 10.1038/cdd.2014.28

[43] Pelisch F, Pozzi B, Risso G, Munoz MJ, Srebrow A. DNA damage-induced heterogeneous nuclear ribonucleoprotein K sumoylation regulates p53 transcriptional activation. The Journal of Biological Chemistry. 2012;**287**:30789-30799. DOI: 10.1074/jbc.M112.390120

[44] Wang B, Tang J, Liao D, Wang G, Zhang M, Sang Y, Cao J, Wu Y, Zhang R, Li S, Ding W, Zhang G, Kang T. Chromobox homolog 4 is correlated with prognosis and tumor cell growth in hepatocellular carcinoma. Annals of Surgical Oncology. 2013;**20**(Suppl 3): S684-S692. DOI: 10.1245/s10434-013-3171-7

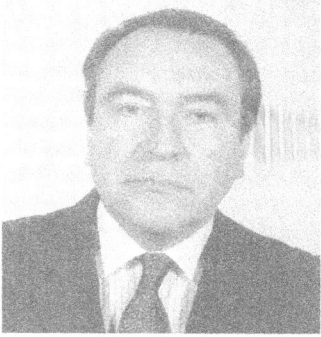

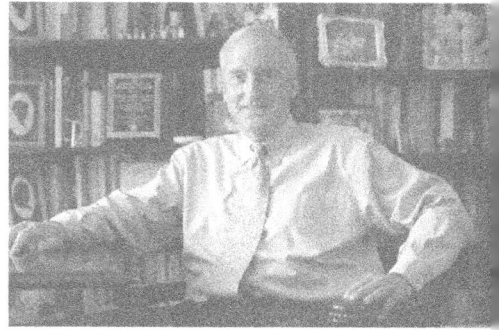

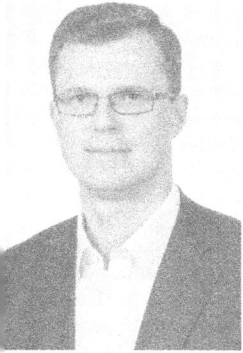

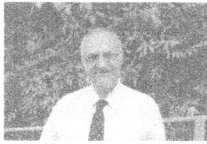

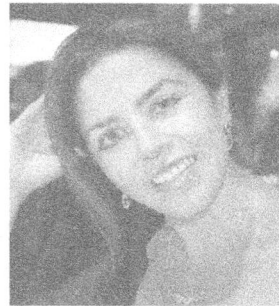

Supporting open minds since 2005

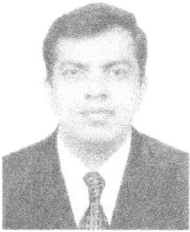

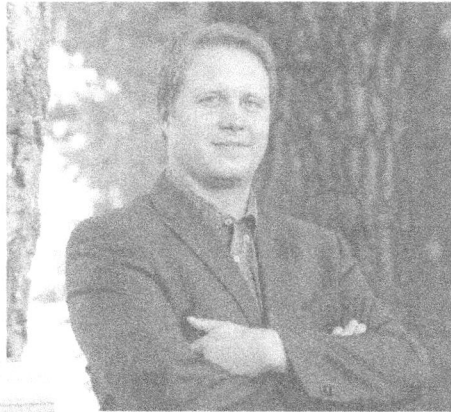

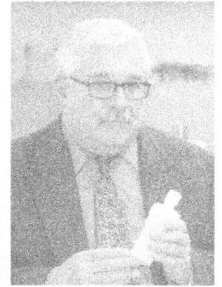

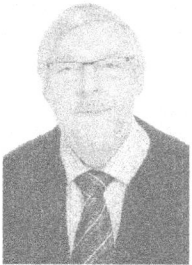

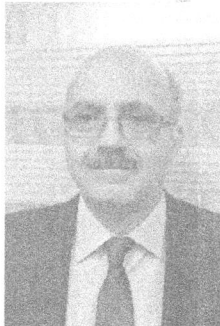

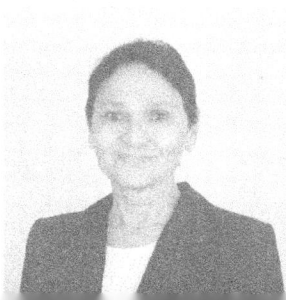

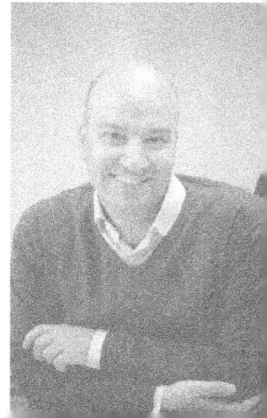

Acupuncture - Resolving Old Controversies and Pointing New Pathways
http://dx.doi.org/10.5772/intechopen.77740
Edited by Marcelo Saad and Roberta de Medeiros

Contributors
Zhiming M. Zhang, Yi-Ning Yin, Jorge E. Quintero, Chuen Heung Yau, Cheuk Long Ip, Mark C. Hou, Ying-Ling Chen, Zhonghua Fu, Dejian Lu, Marcelo Saad, Roberta De Medeiros

Notice
Statements and opinions expressed in the chapters are these of the individual contributors and not necessarily those of the editors or publisher. No responsibility is accepted for the accuracy of information contained in the published chapters. The publisher assumes no responsibility for any damage or injury to persons or property arising out of the use of any materials, instructions, methods or ideas contained in the book.

First published in London, United Kingdom, 2019 by IntechOpen
IntechOpen is the global imprint of INTECHOPEN LIMITED, registered in England and Wales, registration number: 11086078, The Shard, 25th floor, 32 London Bridge Street
London, SE19SG – United Kingdom
Printed in Croatia

British Library Cataloguing-in-Publication Data
A catalogue record for this book is available from the British Library

Additional hard and PDF copies can be obtained from orders@intechopen.com

Acupuncture - Resolving Old Controversies and Pointing New Pathways
Edited by Marcelo Saad and Roberta de Medeiros
p. cm.
Print ISBN 978-1-78984-079-7
Online ISBN 978-1-78984-080-3
eBook (PDF) ISBN 978-1-78984-721-5

We are IntechOpen,
the world's leading publisher of
Open Access books
Built by scientists, for scientists

4,400+
Open access books available

117,000+
International authors and editors

130M+
Downloads

Our authors are among the

151
Countries delivered to

Top 1%
most cited scientists

12.2%
Contributors from top 500 universities

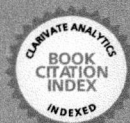

Interested in publishing with us?
Contact book.department@intechopen.com

Numbers displayed above are based on latest data collected.
For more information visit www.intechopen.com

Meet the editors

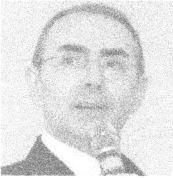

Marcelo Saad, MD, PhD (Brazil), is a physician, board certified in acupuncture. He has a doctorate in the Sciences of Rehabilitation from the Federal University of S. Paulo. He is also current director member of the Spiritist-Medical Association of S. Paulo. He has been invited to the upcoming postgraduate course in Interfaith Hospital Chaplaincy, Santa Marcelina Medical School. Besides his work as a medical acupuncturist in private practice, he is also engaged in scientific publications, editorial collaborations with journals and books, medical lectures, and participation in scholarly tasks. His main interests are religiosity in healthcare, acupuncture, and complementary therapies.

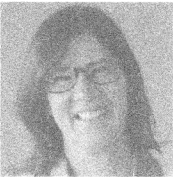

Roberta de Medeiros, PhD (Brazil), is a biologist and holds a doctorate in Comparative Physiology from Universidade Estadual Paulista. She has experience in teaching and research of neurophysiology and human physiology both in graduate (medicine, biomedicine, nutrition, physiotherapy, and occupational therapy) and in postgraduate courses. As well as being a full professor of human physiology at Centro Universitario S. Camilo, she also teaches in special programs for other universities. Her main research field is neural plasticity, but recently she has dedicated herself to the study of all factors related to health preservation.

Contents

Preface

Acupuncture may have about 4000 years of history, but it has only been clinically accepted in the West for some 40 years. Acupuncture receives both praise from its users and skepticism from its critics. High-quality scientific studies have advanced, but the technique in health services has stagnated. In this current scenario of contrasts, *Acupuncture–Resolving Old Controversies and Pointing New Pathways* intends to be a modern reference for scholars, without totally exhausting the subject. The editors expect this work to assist with the advancement of the scientific understanding and clinical usage of acupuncture. The authors are well versed in the subject and, along with literature reviews, are able to add their own impressions.

In this book, some traditional fundamentals of ancient Asian medicine are translated into the current scientific knowledge of neurophysiology and mechanisms of action. Specific variations of acupuncture, such as the scalp microsystem technique, are discussed and explained. Practical aspects, such as education on acupuncture, are enriched with descriptions of novel treatments. The therapeutic use of acupuncture and related techniques is explored regarding their incorporation into a comprehensive integrative medicine approach.

The chapter "Acupuncture—What Controversies? What Pathways?" (by the editors) introduces the reader to the nature and purpose of the book, as well as the significance of its contents for readers. The editors describe the clash between strengths and weaknesses (the controversies) of acupuncture as if it were a game. At the same time, they discuss the strategies (pathways) to keep this game going.

The chapter "Functional Imaging and Physiological Modulation with Acupuncture in Parkinson's Disease and Nonhuman Primate Models of Dopamine Dysfunction" (Zhiming M. Zhang, Jorge E. Quintero, and Yi-Ning Yin) explores the neuropathology of Parkinson's disease and physiological modulation with acupuncture in a model in rhesus monkeys. It is a source of in-depth knowledge about the neuropathology of Parkinson's disease, a description of findings in animal models with this disease, and a documentary of effects of acupuncture on this condition. The unprecedented information makes this manuscript unique and the high level of detail has the potential to advance the treatment of this disease with acupuncture.

The chapter "Fu's Subcutaneous Needling: A Novel Therapeutic Proposal" (Zhonghua Fu and Dejian Lu) reports on an acupuncture system developed and tested by the authors for more than 22 years. The text is well detailed, covering all the complexities of the system: its peculiar terminology, the specially developed needle, the needling and manipulation technique, and the clinical indications. All this is presented in an objective topical format, with very informative figures.

The chapter "Scalp Acupuncture and Mental Disorders" (Chuen Heung Yau and Cheuk Long Ip) is a very comprehensive review of the scientific literature on scalp acupuncture in the treatment of mental diseases. The text covers the history of the procedure, the modern direction for mental disorders, the assumed mechanisms of action, and the limitations of current knowledge due to the paucity of research.

In addition, clinical utility is explored with a description of procedure routines, strategic planning with acupoint selection, indications for which mental disorders may benefit, and contraindications of the procedure.

The chapter "Ultrasound Detection Acupuncture Needling Training: Description of the Method" (Mark C. Hou and Ying-Ling Chen) describes a training method for acupuncture point needling with ultrasound guidance. The method is detailed in a scientifically correct manner, in addition to the evaluation of the training stages. The clinical relevance of this matter is the potential to reduce adverse effects and to inspire other services to adopt such routines.

As editors, we thank the contributing authors for their exquisite work, and we congratulate IntechOpen for its efforts in book production. For you, the readers, we hope to match the trust you put in this work, and we hope you find it useful.

Marcelo Saad, MD, PhD
Director Member at the Spiritist Medical Association,
S. Paulo (SP), Brazil

Roberta de Medeiros, PhD
Full Professor of Physiology,
Centro Universitário S. Camilo,
S. Paulo (SP), Brazil

Chapter 1

Introductory Chapter: Acupuncture - What Controversies? What Pathways?

Marcelo Saad and Roberta de Medeiros

1. A constant board game

This is a short chapter, with intention to be introductory for the nature and purpose of the book subject matter, as well as the significance of its contents for the readers. The field of acupuncture as a scientifically accepted therapy in the West is constantly evolving. All proponents of acupuncture are well convinced of the value of this therapy, and they are quite satisfied with the current documentation regarding its safety, efficiency, effectiveness, and cost-benefit ratio [1]. However, there are still many gaps on this knowledge, equally evidenced in the scholar literature. Very often, proponents of acupuncture have to justify all over again and again their point to the academic-scientific community, since critics are always remembering the flaws.

This duality looks like the antagonism in a board game, represented by the clash between the positive and negative aspects of the technique. In this analogy, the pieces of both sides are in a continuous struggle between the forces strengthening the validity of acupuncture and the movements reducing its legitimacy (**Figure 1**). The positive aspects include everything science recognizes and endorses objectively, added to everything the patients who use the technique feel subjectively. The negative aspects include everything acupuncture is objectively owing to science while researches do not provide all the answers, added to everything subjectively derived from prejudice and ignorance against this technique.

Following this analogy, the new pathways are represented by the strategies the proponents of acupuncture will use to strengthen their arguments and weaken the detractors' arguments, to advance beyond this standoff. This chapter will put the reader on the position of a player interested on the acupuncture advancement. The adversary is virtual, embodying all the closed minds focused only on the acupuncture frailties. To win any game, the player must know his own strengths as well as his own weaknesses. Then, the player will identify threats and opportunities on the distribution of pieces along the board. Finally, he will work to keep the maximum amount of pieces, at the same time eliminating the opponent pieces. The lines below will discourse about intriguing this game.

2. The pieces on our part of the board

2.1 A millenary tradition

The longevity of acupuncture already speaks enough for itself. Acupuncture and correlated techniques have been practiced in China and other Asian countries for millennia. The generally accepted history of acupuncture in China can be

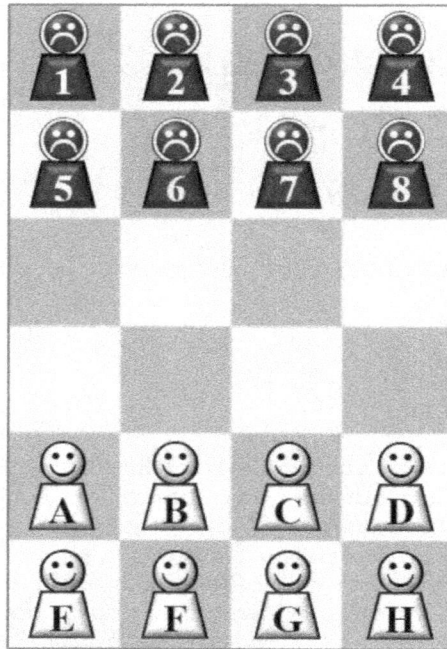

Figure 1.
This board game is an allegory on the constant clash between the elements that sustain acupuncture (the white pieces, on the first-person player's side) and the weaknesses that destabilize acupuncture (the black pieces, on the side of the opponent).

traced back at least 3000 years (the sources diverge, some cites 4000 years), when rudimentary stone needles were used. Besides these archeological clues, the earliest recorded mention of acupuncture is on the classic Yellow Emperor's Inner Classic, written on the second century B.C. Currently, it is routinely practiced in China, Japan, Korea, Hong Kong, and Taiwan as part of the whole healthcare system.

2.2 Worldwide diffusion and acceptance

Acupuncture arrived in Europe in the seventeenth century through the contact of Christian missionaries and European merchants with the Chinese. A resurgent interest among clinicians came only by the nineteenth century in Britain, France, and Germany, when acupuncture arrived also to North America. However, the advances of standard medicine and biological sciences have marginalized acupuncture, and this technique was almost restricted to the Eastern districts of large cities. Acupuncture has gained popularity in the media just about 40 years ago. While in China in 1971, James Reston, a famous journalist and vice president of the New York Times, had an acute appendicitis. Chinese physicians performed an emergency appendectomy, and his postoperative pain was relieved by acupuncture. Reston reported his experience in an historical article in his newspaper [2]. This fact brought great publicity to acupuncture and renewed Western interest in this form of treatment.

2.3 Scientific acceptance through the front door

Scientific publication on acupuncture grew slowly from the 1970s and quickly increased in the last few decades. Some milestones are noteworthy: the

North American National Institutes of Health Consensus Development Panel on Acupuncture, published in 1998 [3], and the World Health Organization (WHO) Review and Analysis of Reports on Controlled Clinical Trials, in 2002 [4]. Today, an extensive bibliography supports the appropriateness of acupuncture use for many defined clinical conditions. Both efficacy and effectiveness of acupuncture have been examined through research with strong methodology. Efficacy is a concept related to mechanisms of action, mainly the effects beyond the placebo. Efficacy measures the impact of an intervention on outcome in ideal conditions, with an emphasis on controlling for placebo effects. Effectiveness is related to how something works in clinical healthcare. This real-world benefit is a measure of the overall impact of an intervention on outcome, as would be expected in routine care. Some trials attempting to address the questions of efficacy and effectiveness are designed with three arms, including true acupuncture, sham procedure, and a comparison treatment.

2.4 East and West can learn with each other

The integration of this strange needling therapy was facilitated with the concept of "Western Medical Acupuncture," a method of peripheral neural stimulation, adapting the Chinese tradition to the knowledge of physiology and other sciences. In such approach, the classic acupoints are selected considering the best places to stimulate the nervous system, inducing local and distant reflexes and neuromodulation. Old and new approaches need not to be mutually exclusive, since modern Western ideas can complement Eastern millennial wisdom. The Eastern thought has holistic views, nonlinear logic, and empirical observation. The Western reasoning is based on reductionist theories, linear causalities, and scientific endorsement. If opposites attract themselves, this can be a perfect marriage [5].

2.5 Multi-institutional acknowledgement of acupuncture

Since 1979, the WHO has proclaimed acupuncture as a clinical practice. In 1996, the North American Food and Drug Administration (FDA) reclassified the needles to a category of accepted medical instruments. In Brazil, acupuncture is officially recognized as a medical specialty since 1995. In the United Kingdom, acupuncture is used in many National Health Service general practices, as well as the majority of pain clinics and hospices. In 2010, the United Nations Educational, Scientific and Cultural Organization (UNESCO) decreed acupuncture as Intangible Cultural Heritage of Humanity. The World Federation of Acupuncture-Moxibustion Societies is currently one of the non-state actors in official relations with the WHO.

2.6 A respectable complementary therapy (CT)

A CT is a procedure used along with standard treatments, although it is not considered orthodox. On the other hand, an alternative therapy is used instead of standard treatments, which is not the best medical practice. In the last decades, acupuncture left the category of a suspect doubtful alternative therapy to become a respectable complementary therapy. Acupuncture can be offered in full compatibility with conventional treatment, because no conceptual conflict surges if they are simultaneously used. This characteristic is different from some alternative therapies, in which some paradigm conflict with conventional treatment, and even sometimes demands its abandonment. This appraisal boosts acupuncture to figure among treatment options in clinical guidelines for many conditions [6].

2.7 An advantageous treatment in many senses

Respecting the indications and contraindications, the combination of acupuncture with conventional resources tends to lead to more complete and long-lasting results [7]. An important factor for such acceptance is acupuncture is a relatively safe technique. Acupuncture is a minimally invasive procedure with good risk-benefit ratio. Acupuncture is suitable for almost all people (including children), with few exceptions in very specific conditions. Potential harm is generally restricted to minor adverse effects, such as pain at needling site, bruises, drowsiness, and skin irritation. Major harm is rarely reported, and most serious adverse events appear to be related to negligence, recklessness, and/or malpractice.

2.8 *Vox populi, vox Dei* (the voice of the people is the voice of God)

Despite the astonishing advancements of conventional medicine and technology in the last decades, there was also a parallel growing interest in complementary therapies among many people [8]. More and more patients express their desire to consume less medication, as they say pharmacological approach has limited results, many side effects, and high cost. The clinician really engaged on a real patient-centered care has to be updated with modern developments on acupuncture. The contemporary concept of integrative medicine is a healthcare approach that partners the patient and the clinician on a healing journey. This is done through the appropriate use of both conventional and complementary techniques. The priority of this combination is to use, whenever possible, natural and less invasive interventions, provided they are safe and worthy. Such comprehensive approach takes selectively the most beneficial effects from different disciplines; at the same time, it meets the patient's values.

3. The pieces of the adversary

3.1 Acupuncture and TCM are "not to be sold separately"

Acupuncture was validated by conventional science separately from the traditional Chinese medicine (TCM). This oriental medicine is a coherent system to promote health and treat disease. Its resources, besides acupuncture, include lifestyle modification (e.g., Chinese diet therapy), herbal therapy, mind-body disciplines (e.g., qigong and meditation), physical practices (e.g., breathing exercises and tai chi), and manual therapy (e.g., massage and tui-na). By the way, it is very likely that the other disciplines arose much before acupuncture, being this particular technique an outspread of this major knowledge. Some groups of practitioners claim that it is nonsense to use acupuncture disconnected from a complete TCM approach. One of the arguments is that TCM is eminently a health promotion system, focusing on disease prevention. Thus, it would be a Western misrepresentation to resort to acupuncture only when the patient is ill.

3.2 Classical theory has "mystical" and confused elements

TCM is based on the concept that qi (the putative vital energy) flows along supposed network of meridians through the body. The harmony between natural opposing forces of yin and yang modulates the balance of spiritual, emotional, mental, and physical health. Diagnosis of an unbalance state is based on tongue and pulse parameters. The so-called triple warmer has no correspondence with an organic structure. Ordinary people will have a huge difficulty to understand terms like "fire on the liver." In addition, most practitioners don't speak the same terms for acupoints and meridians, with some using an alphanumeric code and others the transliterations from the Chinese alphabet [9]. The WHO scientific group proposed in 1991 a standard international nomenclature on acupuncture; however, it is adopted more by researches than by practitioners.

3.3 Acupuncture has many and very heterogeneous expressions

There is a dizzying diversity of treatment designs, considering parameters such as number of needles used, the process of acupoint election, the needling technique, the duration of each session, and the weekly frequency of sessions. Besides needling itself, other classical forms of acupoint stimulation include moxibustion (warming), cupping (negative pressure on the skin), pressure (using devices or fingers), gua sha (scraping), and electrostimulation (either over the skin or through a needle). In addition, acupuncture-correlated techniques are other forms of treatment based on the same principles of acupoint stimulation. They include trigger point needling, laser stimulation, injections on acupuncture point, and the myriad of micro-systems (auricular, scalp, hand, foot, among many others). All this diversity of schools confuses the patients and disrupts the comparison of different papers.

3.4 Mechanisms of action are not totally known

Technically speaking, acupuncture is a method of peripheral neural stimulation by puncturing the skin with a needle on specific anatomical points. It promotes changes in the sensory, motor, autonomic, visceral, hormonal, and immune functions. However, just as physicists seek "The Theory of Everything", their Holy Grail, acupuncture has not yet been able to fit in all the pieces of the biological puzzle to explain how the whole works. A plethora of neurophysiological pathways is demonstrated in countless researches of the highest quality. However, each finding generally serves to explain a single specific effect. It is as if we could see one tree at a time but could not get away enough to see the whole forest. This difficulty of interconnecting all the accumulated knowledge prevents researchers to explain the differences between good and bad responders, as well as whether the effects observed on healthy populations can be extrapolated for sick people.

3.5 A notion (albeit false) that placebo is the main effect

A recurrent criticism on studies of acupuncture through randomized trials controlled by placebo is that both the sham and real acupuncture lead to positive effects. The hasty conclusion is acupuncture acts mainly through placebo effect. However, this understanding is not appropriate, since the needling is not the only therapeutic element. The lack of difference between real and sham groups may underestimate the total effect of acupuncture treatment. The randomized clinical trial controlled by placebo was designed to test drugs, considering only its pharmacological effects. On acupuncture, the physiological component is intertwined to the non-biological processes, and both can be equally important [10]. The environment in acupuncture (already beginning on anamnesis) surely amplifies the extension of the physiological effects. This limitation to design a research is worsened by an insufficient improvement of placebo models. Attempts for placebo acupuncture could be using a false (sham) acupoint, a superficial puncture (with skin perforation), or a simulated needle insertion (without skin perforation) using a blunt device. All of them can produce false-positive results.

3.6 Professional competencies are not universally standardized

Questions about the competency to practice acupuncture are discussed world-wide. Today, each country has its local legislation to assign who is allowed to perform acupuncture. Sometimes, anyone with some qualifications or experience is allowed to be called acupuncturist, even people without formal graduation in a healthcare course. In these cases, the practitioner receives education only focusing on acupuncture and/or TCM, and acupuncture will be offered outside a clinical environment. The risk of diagnosis or treatment delay, due to symptoms masking on a serious disease, is increased if clinical red flags are ignored [11]. The patient protection must be the priority when deciding on training standards and licensure requirements for practitioners. In acupuncture, clinical results vary with the level of training and the length of experience of the practitioner.

3.7 A treatment for a few open-minded people

In our consumerist society, most clients seek immediate solutions for their health problems. Compared to drug treatment, acupuncture may seem a boring, tardy, and expensive option to many people. The treatment with acupuncture typically involves several sessions and follow-up, which may be inconvenient for some patients. Many times, a private treatment has to be paid out-of-pocket, when it is not covered by health insurance policies. The cost of a course of sessions varies widely between providers, and the whole treatment can be expensive. Furthermore, it is unpredictable what will happen when the patient reduces the sessions' frequency or stops the treatment. Patients have to be adequately informed on what to expect, in order to be motivated by realistic prospects. They also must understand that the effectiveness of acupuncture cannot be generalized, as its effect varies largely from patient to patient.

3.8 Rejection by a part of clinicians

Some clinicians state they find no reason to indicate stranger therapeutic systems, since the value and success of conventional biomedical science are just enough. For clinicians who think so, having to learn the principles and indications of other practices would be an unnecessary task. Such colleagues would indicate acupuncture only when they have no further resources to offer (or even when they want to get rid of the patient, etc.). In some cases, disregarding acupuncture is actually an excuse (conscious or unconscious) for lack of time (or commitment) to explore everything that could be beneficial to the patient.

4. In short

As the game goes on, acupuncture needs to prove on a daily basis that it has nothing to do with other picturesque therapies. A lot of energy must be spent to unstick acupuncture of weird East prescriptions such as the powder of rhinoceros' horn, a useless pinch of keratin that is leading this animal to extinction. However, this is a fact: acupuncture came to stay. The opposition to this therapeutic modality would never eliminate it from the canon of good complementary therapies. However, such opposition can clutter many advances for acupuncture use, from no inclusion in clinical guidelines to limitation for reimbursement to health insurance users. More slowly than we would like, the score of this game hangs to the side of the fittest player. It's up to us to continue this game, even though it may not have an end. Anyway, every little advance is a victory.

Author details

Marcelo Saad[1*] and Roberta de Medeiros[2]

1 Spiritist Medical Association of S. Paulo, S. Paulo, SP, Brazil

2 Centro Universitário S. Camilo, S. Paulo, SP, Brazil

*Address all correspondence to: msaad@uol.com.br

IntechOpen

References

[1] Saad M, Jorge LL, Vieira MSR, de Medeiros R. Integration of acupuncture for outpatients and inpatients in a general hospital in Brazil. Acupuncture in Medicine. 2009;**27**(4):178-179. DOI: 10.1136/aim.2009.001446

[2] Reston J. Now, About My Operation in Peking. New York Times. July 26:1. 1971. Retrieved from: http://select. nytimes.com/gst/abstract.html?res=FB0 D11FA395C1A7493C4AB178CD85F4587 85F9 [Accessed: April 16, 2019]

[3] NIH Consensus Conference. Acupuncture. JAMA. 1998;**280**(17): 1518-1524. Retrieved from: http://www. ncbi.nlm.nih.gov/pubmed/9809733 [Accessed: April 16, 2019]

[4] WHO. Acupuncture-Review and Analysis of Reports on Controlled Clinical Trials. Geneva, Switzerland: World Health Organization; 2002; 87 pp. Retrieved from: http:// digicollection.org/hss/en/d/Js4926e/ [Accessed April 16, 2019]. ISBN: 92-4-154543-7

[5] Saad M, de Medeiros R. Complementary therapies for fibromyalgia syndrome: A rational approach. Current Pain and Headache Reports. 2013;**17**(8):354. DOI: 10.1007/ s11916-013-0354-7

[6] Birch S, Lee MS, Alraek T, Kim T-H. Overview of treatment guidelines and clinical practical guidelines that recommend the use of acupuncture: A bibliometric analysis. The Journal of Alternative and Complementary Medicine. 2018;**24**(8):752-769. DOI: 10.1089/acm.2018.0092

[7] Saad M, de Medeiros R. Poor results in pain management: Suggestion for how to interpret them. Medical Acupuncture. 2015;**27**(4):247-248. DOI: 10.1089/acu.2015.29005.lte

[8] Jishun J, Mittelman M. Acupuncture: Past, present, and future. Global Advances in Health and Medicine. 2014;**3**(4):6-8. DOI: 10.7453/ gahmj.2014.042

[9] Langevin HM, Wayne PM. What is the point? The problem with acupuncture research that no one wants to talk about. The Journal of Alternative and Complementary Medicine. 2018;**24**(3):200-207. DOI: 10.1089/ acm.2017.0366

[10] de Medeiros R, Saad M. Complementary therapies— Considerations before recommend, tolerate or proscribe them. In: Complementary Therapies for the Contemporary Healthcare. Rijeka, Croatia: InTech Publisher; 2012. DOI: 10.5772/50446

[11] Saad M. Why medical acupuncture? Medical Acupuncture. 2009;**21**(4):291-291. DOI: 10.1089/acu.2009.2005

Functional Imaging and Physiological Modulation with Acupuncture in Parkinson's Disease and Nonhuman Primate Models of Dopamine Dysfunction

Yi-Ning Yin, Jorge E. Quintero and Zhiming M. Zhang

Abstract

Here we review functional imaging and neurophysiological evidence for the pre-clinical and clinical use of electroacupuncture, a non-pharmaceutical-based thera-peutic strategy, to relieve parkinsonian symptoms. Outcomes from those studies provide evidence that the effect of electroacupuncture can be objectively measured in nonhuman primate models of Parkinson's disease and in patients with Parkinson's disease. In addition, the evidence continues to support that electroacupuncture can be used in preclinical and clinical studies simply, safely, and effectively as an alternative and complementary treatment for disorders in Parkinson's disease.

Keywords: acupuncture, pharmacological MRI, glutamate, cortex, electrochemistry

1. Introduction

Acupuncture has been gaining popularity for treatment of various disorders as an alternative therapy and has been used for years as treatment for a wide range of ailments from lower back pain to stroke to osteoarthritis to Parkinson's disease (PD) [1–5]. Classical acupuncture is based on 14 mapped main channels on the body with about 365 acupoints distributed on the channels (meridian system); the flow of Qi (the vital life force or "energy") maintains the balance and harmony of Yin and Yang. Any blockage of these channels or abnormal movement of Qi will result in ill-ness, and acupuncture, by stimulating these acupoints along the meridian channels with needles, helps to restore movement of the Qi and Qi homeostasis (De Qi), thus modulating the autonomic nervous system and relieving the symptoms of various illnesses [6, 7]. The underlying mechanism of acupuncture has been under intense investigation and many theories have been discussed in the scientific community. For example, connective tissues or perivascular space with decreased electrical impedance and increased electrical conductivity have been suggested to constitute the meridian channels with acupoints along the pathway [7, 8]. Nevertheless, the efficacy of acupuncture remains largely unclear because of a skeptical attitude of how acupuncture works (especially within the framework of Western Medicine), methodological flaws, and an absence of rigorous studies using objective outcome measures [1]. To date, the clinical outcomes of acupuncture are assessed by empirical observations rather than by objective, quality analysis [1, 3, 5].

Recent, rapid advances in technology, especially the use of functional magnetic resonance imaging (fMRI) to map global and/or target-specific bran regions, have shown great promise and could be extremely helpful for acupuncture studies in human subjects when combined with subjective measurements [8]. Pharmacological MRI (phMRI), a new application of fMRI, is using fMRI methods to map drug-induced activations inside the brain [9]. In this chapter, we discuss how phMRI can be used to map dopaminergic drug-induced changes in the brain before and after acupuncture treatment in parkinsonian monkeys. Similarly, fMRI methods have been used in the PD clinic. As an example, with acute acupuncture stimulations at GB34, analysis of fMRI signals showed activations in the putamen and the primary motor cortex, and these activations induced by acupuncture were correlated with patient self-reported improvements of finger-tapping [10]. Furthermore, phMRI has been used to monitor other treatments associated with PD in a preclinical, translational study [11]. The utility of fMRI/phMRI has even been extended to differentiate dysfunction in the basal ganglia between parkinsonian and aged monkeys [12]. Based on those clinical and preclinical studies, these imaging modalities have the possibility to help untangle the underlying neural mechanisms of acupuncture.

To date, few studies have been conducted *in vivo* to directly investigate the relationship between acute acupuncture stimulation and its effects on modulating neurotransmitters especially in large animals such as the rhesus macaque. In this chapter, to our knowledge, we would be the first to begin exploring whether acupuncture stimulation could suppress, or activate, cortical glutamate in normal and PD monkeys. In addition, we will also review fMRI and phMRI studies to provide some direct evidence demonstrating the relationship between acupuncture and neuronal activity and changes in neurotransmitter signaling in the CNS.

2. Evidence from neuroimaging studies

2.1 Functional/pharmacological MRI study in nonhuman primates

Over the past two decades, our group has been working to objectively and safely monitor anti-parkinsonian effects and brain activity modulated by electroacupuncture (EA) in nonhuman primates modeling human PD. We maintained a group of late middle aged rhesus monkeys with long-term (>5 years) mild to moderate parkinsonism rendered by our standard procedures, unilateral administration of 1-methyl-4-phenyl-1,2,3,6-tetrahydropyridine (MPTP) [13]. This group of parkinsonian rhesus macaques was extensively evaluated by a computerized behavioral testing battery and by phMRI scans [14, 15]. First, stable parkinsonian features were observed in all animals before entering the EA study and all animals showed positive responses to a levodopa (L-dopa) challenge [14]. phMRI activation was then analyzed by our standard procedure. Briefly, while undergoing fMRI scans, animals received a subcutaneous injection of the dopamine agonist, apomorphine (APO). This pharmacological challenge then serves as the basis for assessing the changes in fMRI responses. Second, the phMRI results revealed that compared with the normal, pre-MPTP, status, APO-induced activations were found in all measured ROIs (**Figure 1A** and **B**, **Table 1**, described in [14]). The differences between normal and post-MPTP stages in response to the apomorphine challenge were significant ($P < 0.001$), especially in the caudate nucleus, putamen, primary motor cortex

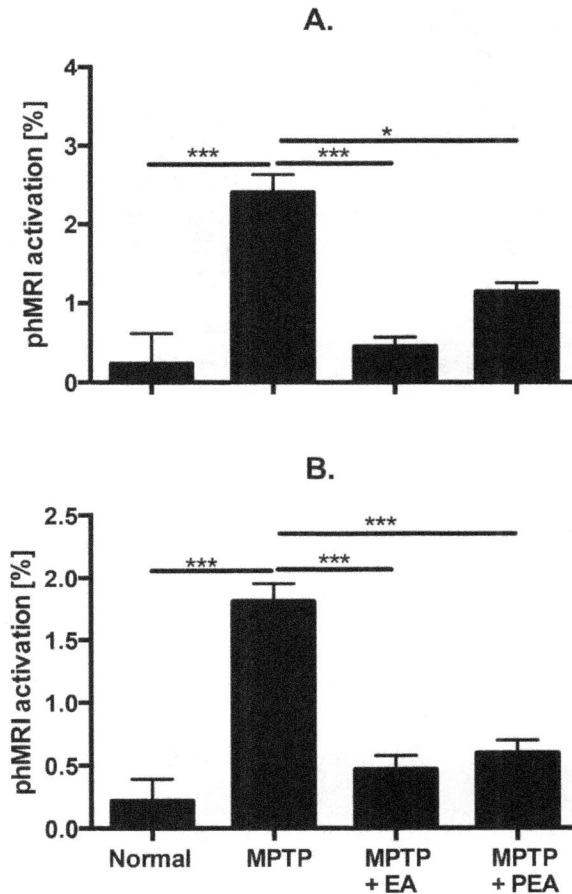

Figure 1.
phMRI activation changes of animals following different treatments. phMRI activation changes of caudate nucleus (A) and putamen (B) following MPTP administration, chronic EA treatment or post EA treatment (from [14]).

(M1), cingulate gyrus and globus pallidus externa (GPe). In contrast, blood oxygen level dependent (BOLD) responses in the pre-motor areas and the globus pallidus interna (GPi) were not significantly different (**Table 1**). These findings were in line with previous results [16] that APO-induced activations were seen in the striatum after animals became parkinsonian. In addition to those responses described above, APO-induced activations were also observed in the MPTP-lesioned primary motor cortex and cingulate gyrus (**Figure 2** and **Table 1**).

The chronic EA treatment appeared to alter neuronal activities in some examined areas such as the caudate nucleus, putamen, primary motor cortex, cingulate gyrus and GPe in which strong APO-evoked activations were initially observed after MPTP lesions but then were significantly reduced after the EA treatment. In some cases, the BOLD activations nearly returned to the levels seen in the normal (pre-lesion) stage (**Figure 1A** and **B** and **Table 1**). However, the phMRI responses were relatively mild in the pre-motor cortex and GPi (**Table 1**). As shown in **Figures 1** and **2**, the most affected regions were the caudate nucleus and primary motor cortex. For example, the APO-induced activations were reduced more than 5-fold in the caudate nucleus and 4-fold in the primary motor cortex. Interestingly,

ROIs	Cingulate	GPe	GPi
Normal	0.74 ± 0.25	−0.27 ± 0.3	−0.16 ± 0.26
MPTP	2.16 ± 0.09[a]	1.92 ± 0.13[a]	0.84 ± 0.41
MPTP + EA	0.58 ± 0.23[b]	0.54 ± 0.19[d,e]	0.44 ± 0.31
MPTP + PEA	0.85 ± 0.11[c]	0.69 ± 0.09[f]	1.11 ± 0.14[d]

GPe, globus pallidus externa; GPi, globus pallidus interna; ROIs, region of interest; EA, electroacupuncture; PEA, post electroacupuncture (from [14]).
[a]*P < 0.001 vs. normal.*
[b]*P < 0.001 vs. MPTP.*
[c]*P < 0.001 vs. MPTP + EA.*
[d]*P < 0.05 vs. normal.*
[e]*P < 0.01 vs. MPTP.*
[f]*P < 0.05 vs. MPTP + EA.*

Table 1.
BOLD-responses in some cortical and subcortical areas.

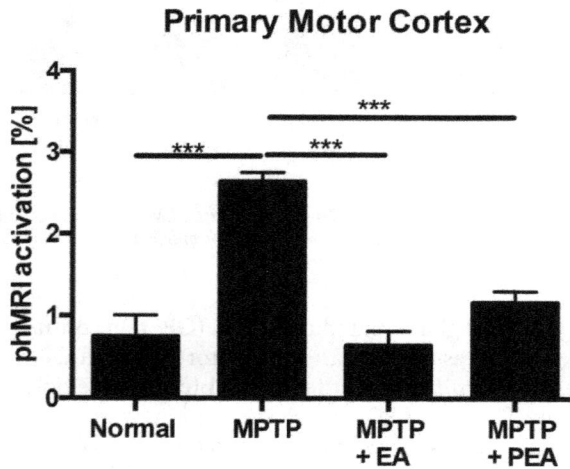

Figure 2.
phMRI activation changes of primary motor cortex following MPTP administration, chronic EA treatment or post EA treatment (adapted from [14]).

residual effects were observed 3 months after the last EA treatment in the caudate nucleus, putamen, primary motor cortex, and cingulate gyrus regions judged by comparing the values of BOLD-activations between MPTP + EA and MPTP + PEA (3 months post EA treatment). A significant difference (P < 0.05) between MPTP + EA and MPTP + PEA was also seen in the GPe (**Table 1**). The results strongly suggest that anti-parkinsonian effects of EA can be objectively assessed, and fMRI/phMRI could be readily translated into the clinic with minor modifications.

2.2 Functional MRI studies in humans

In human studies, acupuncture stimulations that directly modulate brain activity can also be observed [17, 18]. An example of this was carried out by Li and colleagues [17] who used fMRI to investigate the potential neuromechanism of acupuncture on tremor in patients with Parkinson's disease. Li and colleagues compared fMRI signals in patients with Parkinson's disease who were either in the true acupuncture group (TAG) or the sham acupuncture group (SAG). Participants received levodopa for 12 weeks and received the study intervention twice weekly. Participants in TAG were acupunctured on DU20, GB20, and the Chorea-Tremor Controlled Zone. Participants in SAG were given sham acupuncture. fMRI scans of the participant's brains were obtained before and after the 12-week period. As shown in **Figure 3**, acupuncture had specific effects on the activity of the cerebrocerebellar pathways as shown by a decrease in regional homogeneity (ReHo)—an indication of a decrease in local/regional activity. Other measures of brain activity, degree centrality (DC), and amplitude low-frequency fluctuation (ALFF) values, also showed decreases after acupuncture compared to sham. Meanwhile, increased ReHo values were observed within the thalamus and motor cortex [17]. The results of this clinical study demonstrate that functional imaging can directly detect and measure acupuncture-induced brain activities even at the level of the neural network.

In a separate clinic study to examine the underlying mechanisms of acupuncture in patients with major depressive disorders, Wang et al. [19] investigated the resting state functional connectivity (rsFC) in the left and right amygdala before and after verum acupuncture plus the antidepressant fluoxetine versus sham acupuncture plus fluoxetine. Resting-state fMRI data was collected before the first and last treatments. Participants received the study intervention for 8 weeks. Verum acupuncture treatment participants showed (1) greater clinical improvement than sham participants based on the depression rating scales; (2) increased rsFC between the left amygdala and subgenual anterior

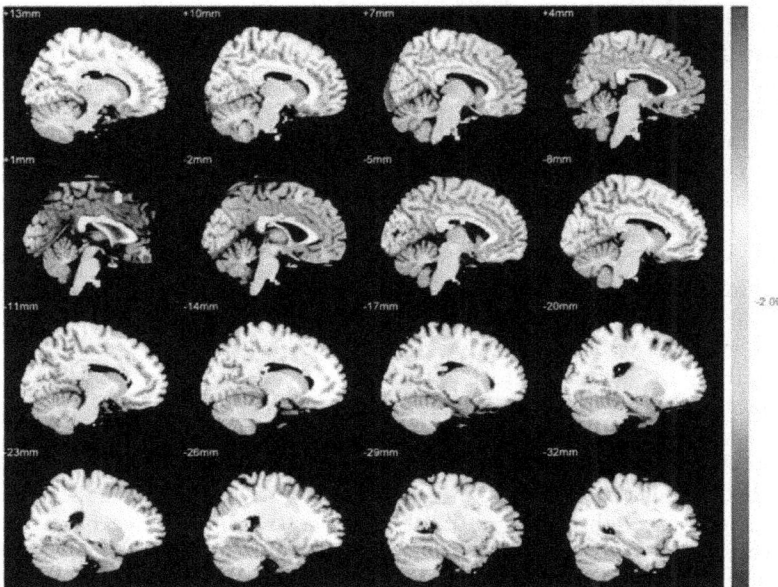

Figure 3.
Differences in ReHo values between the TAG and SAG. (P < 0.05, AlphaSim corrected). Warm colors represent positive ReHo values; blue (cold) colors represent negative ReHo values (from [17]).

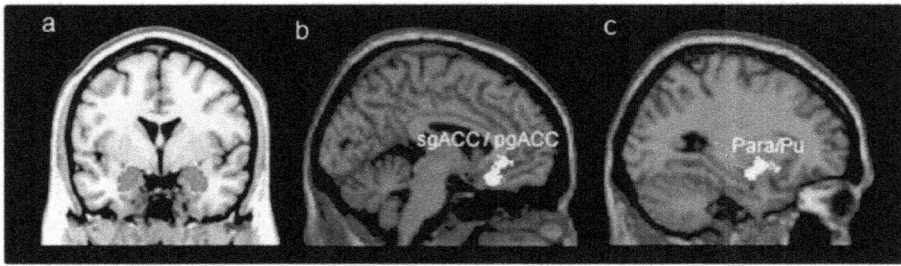

Figure 4.
Amygdala seed locations and brain regions with significant changes (post minus pre) of rsFC with the amygdala (a) modulated by the verum acupuncture plus fluoxetine compared with sham acupuncture plus fluoxetine treatment in the left sgACC/pgACC (b) and left Para/Pu (c). Abbreviations: sgACC, subgenual anterior cingulate cortex; pgACC, pregenual anterior cingulate cortex; Para, parahippocampus; Pu, putamen (from [19]).

cingulate cortex (sgACC)/pregenual anterior cingulate cortex (pgACC); (3) increased rsFC between the right amygdala and left parahippocampus/putamen. And finally, the strength of the amygdala-sgACC/pgACC rsFC was positively associated with a corresponding clinical improvement (**Figure 4**). Their findings show the additive effect of acupuncture to antidepressant treatment and suggest that this effect may be achieved through the limbic system, especially the amygdala and the ACC [19].

3. Evidence from electrochemical studies

In the brain, glutamatergic transmission plays a key role in the normal physiology of those systems that modulate motor activity (especially in the basal ganglia). In Parkinson's disease, glutamatergic transmission is considerably affected particularly in the direct and indirect nigrostriatal pathways, which are known to involve glutamatergic hyperactivity. The glutamatergic hyperactive pattern, through a dual role, may exacerbate PD by first promoting excitotoxic events that contribute to the neurodegenerative process and, secondly, by contributing to the pathophysiology of dyskinesias and motor fluctuations that are associated with the chronic use of levodopa [20]. Since excitotoxicity is a glutamate-receptor-mediated phenomenon, growing interest and work have been dedicated to the research for modulators of glutamate neurotransmission that might enable new therapeutic interventions to slow the neurodegenerative process and ameliorate PD symptoms.

To explore the role of glutamate excitotoxicity in both acupuncture and pathogenesis of PD, we designed a study to address the question of whether changes in cortical glutamate levels were one of the underlying mechanisms of EA (previously unpublished results). Based on human acupuncture studies in patients with PD, we trained two rhesus monkeys with mild but stable parkinsonian features (MPTP-induced) including bradykinesia, rigidity on the affected upper and lower limbs. In addition, stooped posture and mild postural instability were also evident [13]. Then, these animals were treated with chronic (intermittent) EA treatments (3 session/week/4 months) at acupoints ST 36, GB34, or LI 4 (**Figure 5**). Subsequently, they were also studied for behavioral changes by a non-biased, computerized testing battery. Results demonstrated that EA significantly improved motor functions measured by increased movement speed after a 4-month EA treatment (data now shown). Following the last EA treatment and behavioral tests, animals were anesthetized and resting levels of L-glutamate were measured in the primary motor areas (upper body) by enzyme-based biosensors [21] with acute EA stimulation at GV14 + EX-B9 or GV14 + ST 36 or LI 4 on both sides, or GV14 + non-acupoints (**Figure 5**). EA-induced

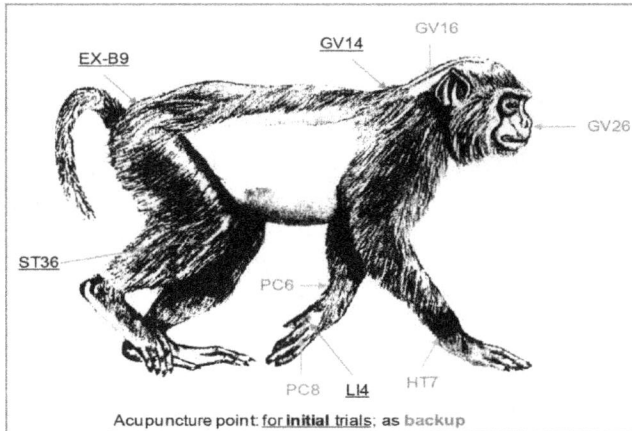

Yao Yi	EX-B9	Epilepsy, headache, insomnia, constipation
Da Zui	GV 14	Cough, neck stiffness, epilepsy
He Gu	LI 4	Headache, epistaxis, deafness, toothache, facial swelling, facial paralysis, sore throat.
Zu San Li	ST 36	Various pain
Shen Men	HT 7	Cardiac pain, irritability, psychosis, epilepsy, poor memory, palpitations, insomnia
Nei Guan	PC 6	Cardiac pain, palpitations, epilepsy, vomiting, contracture and pain of elbow and arm.
Lao Gong	PC8	Cardiac pain, epilepsy.
Feng Fu	GV16	Wind-stroke with aphasia, headache, neck stiffness, eye-dizziness, epistaxis, sore throat, Epilepsy
Shui Gou	GV26	Facial paralysis, facial swelling, Psychosis, epilepsy, loss of consciousness, infantile convulsions, stiffness and pain of lower back.

Figure 5.
Acupuncture points used in the study.

changes in cortical glutamate could be recorded in real time (2 Hz) with glutamate-sensitive biosensors (**Figure 6A**). The EA treatments of GV14 + EX-B9, or GV14 + ST 36 significantly decreased basal levels of glutamate in the primary motor cortex on the hemisphere contralateral to the MPTP-lesion immediately after the stimulator was turned on and returned to baseline levels after it was turned off. By contrast, stimulation of GV14 and a non-acupuncture point produced no fluctuation in basal glutamate activity (**Figure 6B**). These results support the idea that EA can produce transient effects on cortical levels of glutamate that could be a means of providing a potential therapy for PD.

Acupuncture can alter extracellular glutamate as seen in our pilot nonhuman primate study and those results are supported by acupuncture studies in rodents. Lee et al. reported that acupuncture can attenuate extracellular glutamate levels in a global ischemia model in rat. In the study, the authors found that acupuncture at GB34 and GB39 significantly suppressed glutamate function compared to control animals [22]. Later, Kim et al. demonstrated that acupuncture at HT7 can inhibit methamphetamine-induced behaviors, dopamine release and hyperthermia in the nucleus accumbens through the group II metabotropic glutamate receptors [23].

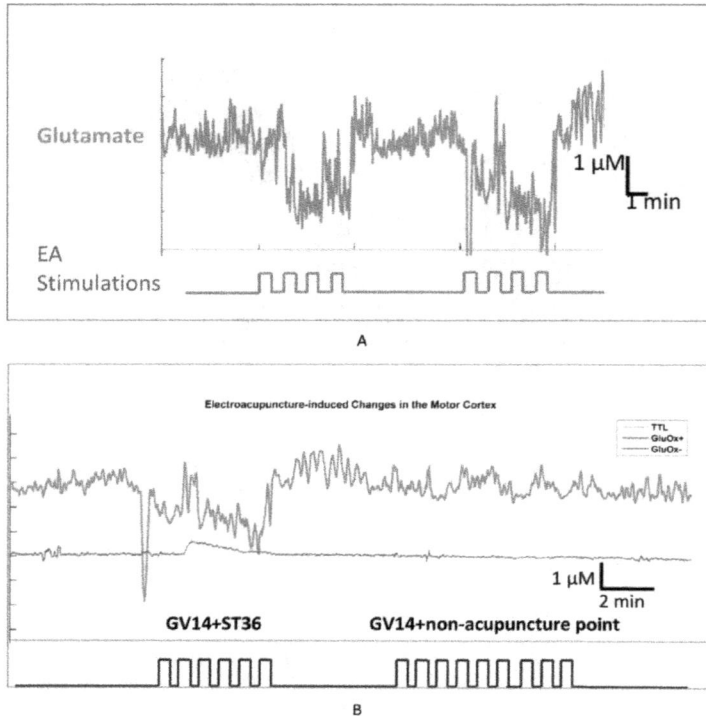

Figure 6.
*(A) Real-time measurements of the basal glutamate change in the motor cortex with and without acupuncture stimulations. Glutamate changes in the unlesioned motor cortex produced by EA stimulation at GV14 + ST36 (right side). Glutamate biosensors were used to measure glutamate levels. One biosensor recording site is coated with glutamate oxidase and capable of detecting glutamate a reference biosensor recording site lacking glutamate oxidase and incapable of detecting glutamate is used to subtract interfering agents. (B) Real-time measurement of the basal glutamate changes in the motor cortex with and without acupuncture stimulations. Glutamate changes in the unlesioned motor cortex produced by EA stimulation at GV14 + ST36 (right side) and GV14 + nonacupuncture points. TTL: transistor-transistor logic (event marker). GluOx+ (biosensor recording site coated with glutamate oxidase and capable of detecting glutamate), GluOx− (biosensor recording site lacking glutamate oxidase and incapable of detecting glutamate). Note the stimulation induced artifact in the reference channel (GluOx− recording site) during the course of stimulation that subsides when EA stimulation is terminated. Zoomed inset of **Figure 6A**.*

4. Evidence from objective behavioral testing

4.1 Objective behavioral testing in preclinical studies

For years, our group has been developing testing methods to objectively measure behavioral changes before and after intermittent EA treatments in parkinsonian monkeys. Recently, we reported that EA-induced improvement of parkinsonism in rhesus macaques can be effectively measured using a non-biased, non-invasive and computerized behavioral testing battery [14]. The battery primarily includes a videotracking system to measure movement speed, an Actical accelerometer to monitor home-cage activity 24 h a day, 7 days a week, and an upper limb movement analysis panel to measure a subject retrieval time [14, 24]. As shown in **Figure 7**, significantly deceased movement speed (A), and home cage activity (B), and longer performance time of the affected hand (C) were found following MPTP administration. The movement speed and fine motor performance time were markedly improved with chronic EA treatment (**Figure 7A** and **C**), and movement speed and fine motor performance times virtually returned to pre-MPTP levels. The cage activity was increased but did not reach statistically significant levels because of large variance (**Figure 7B**). Meanwhile, the fine motor performance time was still

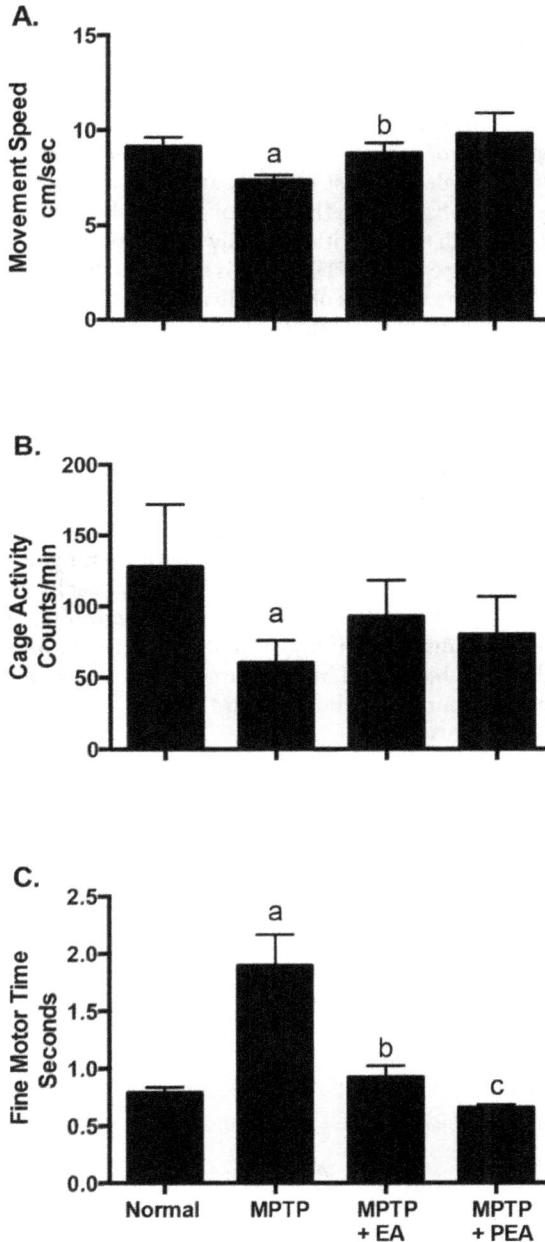

Figure 7.
Behavior changes of animals following different treatments. Movement speed (A), home cage activity (B) and fine motor performance time changes (C) following MPTP administration, chronic EA treatment or post EA treatment (at least 1 months after last EA treatment). (a) P < 0.05 compared with normal; (b) P < 0.05 compared with MPTP; (c) P < 0.05 compared with MPTP + EA (from [14]).

improving one-month post EA treatment (**Figure 7C**). In addition, all animals responded positively to levodopa challenge evident by a 261% increase of home-cage activity measured via Actical counts.

4.2 Objective behavioral testing in clinical studies

In the acupuncture clinic, objective assessments using novel computerized technologies are drawing more attention. Lei and colleagues used body-worn sensor technology in patients with PD to measure a variety of gait parameters [3]. The authors found that EA improved gait function and achieved statistically significant improvements in gait speed under a variety of walking tasks including single-task habitual walking, single-task fast walking, and dual-task fast walking. No significant changes were observed in the control group. Meanwhile, gait improvements were correlated with the activities of daily living component of the Unified Parkinson's Disease Rating Scale (UPDRS). This study further indicates that the effectiveness of EA treatment can be objectively measured and while still used with traditional instruments such as the UPDRS.

5. Summary

Current evidence shows that EA generates measurable changes in the brain that are detectable with functional imaging, behavioral responses, and neurotransmitter signaling. The results from nonhuman primates also provides direct evidence between EA stimulations and dynamic alterations in the resting levels of glutamate in the motor cortex, which may at least partially explain a mechanism of action for EA in the nervous system. Nevertheless, we are only at beginning of a quest to better understand the mechanism of action that underlie acupuncture. The few studies with limited number of subjects will have to expand if we are to understand how acupuncture affects the central nervous system.

Author details

Yi-Ning Yin[1], Jorge E. Quintero[2,3] and Zhiming M. Zhang[2*]

1 Hunter Acupuncture, NSW, Australia

2 Department of Neuroscience, University of Kentucky, Lexington, KY, USA

3 Center for Microelectrode Technology, University of Kentucky, Lexington, KY, USA

*Address all correspondence to: zzhan01@uky.edu

IntechOpen

References

[1] Lee MS, Shin BC, Kong JC, Ernst E. Effectiveness of acupuncture for Parkinson's disease: A systematic review. Movement Disorders. 2008;**23**(11):1505-1515

[2] Lee SJ, Lyu YS, Kang HW, Sohn IC, Koo S, Kim MS, et al. Antinociception of heterotopic electro-acupuncture mediated by the dorsolateral funiculus. The American Journal of Chinese Medicine. 2007;**35**(2):251-264

[3] Lei H, Toosizadeh N, Schwenk M, Sherman S, Karp S, Sternberg E, et al. A pilot clinical trial to objectively assess the efficacy of electroacupuncture on gait in patients with Parkinson's disease using body worn sensors. PLoS One. 2016;**11**(5):e0155613

[4] Rajendran PR, Thompson RE, Reich SG. The use of alternative therapies by patients with Parkinson's disease. Neurology. 2001;**57**(5):790-794

[5] Shulman LM, Wen X, Weiner WJ, Bateman D, Minagar A, Duncan R, et al. Acupuncture therapy for the symptoms of Parkinson's disease. Movement Disorders. 2002;**17**(4):799-802

[6] Li QQ, Shi GX, Xu Q, Wang J, Liu CZ, Wang LP. Acupuncture effect and central autonomic regulation. Evidence-based Complementary and Alternative Medicine. 2013;**2013**:267959

[7] Ma W, Tong H, Xu W, Hu J, Liu N, Li H, et al. Perivascular space: Possible anatomical substrate for the meridian. Journal of Alternative and Complementary Medicine. 2003;**9**(6):851-859

[8] Jia J, Yu Y, Deng JH, Robinson N, Bovey M, Cui YH, et al. A review of Omics research in acupuncture: The relevance and future prospects for understanding the nature of meridians and acupoints. Journal of Ethnopharmacology. 2012;**140**(3):594-603

[9] Leslie RA, James MF. Pharmacological magnetic resonance imaging: A new application for functional MRI. Trends in Pharmacological Sciences. 2000;**21**(8):314-318

[10] Chae Y, Lee H, Kim H, Kim CH, Chang DI, Kim KM, et al. Parsing brain activity associated with acupuncture treatment in Parkinson's diseases. Movement Disorders. 2009;**24**(12):1794-1802

[11] Luan L, Ding F, Ai Y, Andersen A, Hardy P, Forman E, et al. Pharmacological MRI (phMRI) monitoring of treatment in hemiparkinsonian rhesus monkeys. Cell Transplantation. 2008;**17**(4):417-425

[12] Andersen AH, Hardy PA, Forman E, Gerhardt GA, Gash DM, Grondin RC, et al. Pharmacologic MRI (phMRI) as a tool to differentiate Parkinson's disease-related from age-related changes in basal ganglia function. Neurobiology of Aging. 2015;**36**(2):1174-1182

[13] Ding F, Luan L, Ai Y, Walton A, Gerhardt GA, Gash DM, et al. Development of a stable, early stage unilateral model of Parkinson's disease in middle-aged rhesus monkeys. Experimental Neurology. 2008;**212**(2):431-439

[14] Zhang R, Andersen AH, Hardy PA, Forman E, Evans A, Ai Y, et al. Objectively measuring effects of electro-acupuncture in parkinsonian rhesus monkeys. Brain Research. 2018;**1678**:12-19

[15] Zhao F, Fan X, Grondin R, Edwards R, Forman E, Moorehead J, et al. Improved methods

for electroacupuncture and electromyographic recordings in normal and parkinsonian rhesus monkeys. Journal of Neuroscience Methods. 2010;**192**(2):199-206

[16] Zhang Z, Andersen AH, Ai Y, Loveland A, Hardy PA, Gerhardt GA, et al. Assessing nigrostriatal dysfunctions by pharmacological MRI in parkinsonian rhesus macaques. NeuroImage. 2006;**33**(2):636-643

[17] Li Z, Chen J, Cheng J, Huang S, Hu Y, Wu Y, et al. Acupuncture modulates the cerebello-thalamo-cortical circuit and cognitive brain regions in patients of Parkinson's disease with tremor. Frontiers in Aging Neuroscience. 2018;**10**:206

[18] Xiao D. Acupuncture for Parkinson's disease: A review of clinical, animal, and functional magnetic resonance imaging studies. Journal of Traditional Chinese Medicine. 2015;**35**(6):709-717

[19] Wang X, Wang Z, Liu J, Chen J, Liu X, Nie G, et al. Repeated acupuncture treatments modulate amygdala resting state functional connectivity of depressive patients. NeuroImage: Clinical. 2016;**12**:746-752

[20] Ambrosi G, Cerri S, Blandini F. A further update on the role of excitotoxicity in the pathogenesis of Parkinson's disease. Journal of Neural Transmission (Vienna). 2014;**121**(8):849-859

[21] Quintero JE, Day BK, Zhang Z, Grondin R, Stephens ML, Huettl P, et al. Amperometric measures of age-related changes in glutamate regulation in the cortex of rhesus monkeys. Experimental Neurology. 2007;**208**(2):238-246

[22] Lee GJ, Yin CS, Choi SK, Choi S, Yang JS, Lee H, et al. Acupuncture attenuates extracellular glutamate level in global ischemia model of rat.

Neurological Research. 2010;**32** (Suppl 1):79-83

[23] Kim NJ, Ryu Y, Lee BH, Chang S, Fan Y, Gwak YS, et al. Acupuncture inhibition of methamphetamine-induced behaviors, dopamine release and hyperthermia in the nucleus accumbens: Mediation of group II mGluR. Addiction Biology. 2018. DOI: 10.1111/adb.12587

[24] Zhang Z, Andersen A, Smith C, Grondin R, Gerhardt G, Gash D. Motor slowing and parkinsonian signs in aging rhesus monkeys mirror human aging. The Journals of Gerontology. Series A, Biological Sciences and Medical Sciences. 2000;**55**(10):B473-B480

Chapter 3

Fu's Subcutaneous Needling: A Novel Therapeutic Proposal

Zhonghua Fu and Dejian Lu

Abstract

Fu's subcutaneous needling (FSN) uses disposable FSN acupuncture needle as its tool to stimulate the subcutaneous layer by doing horizontal sweeping manipulation. Needling sites are mainly selected around or near tightened muscles which contain one or several myofascial trigger points and cause pain or other illnesses. FSN therapy is originated from classics and based on clinical practice. Out of inheritance and innovation, it is the scientific research achievement of Fu Zhonghua and his research team over 22 years of hard work. It is the original and innovative technology with independent intellectual property rights. FSN therapy is safe, nontoxic, and has no side effect. This chapter is drafted in order to facilitate clinical study and application, by which the terms and definitions, indications and contraindications, operating procedures, exceptions, and the relative handling as well as precautions are written down.

Keywords: Fu's subcutaneous needling (FSN), FSN therapy, tightened muscle (TM), insertion point, sweeping movement, reperfusion approach

1. Terminology and definition

The following terms and definitions apply to this standard.

1.1 Fu's subcutaneous needling

Fu's subcutaneous needling (FSN) uses disposable FSN acupuncture needle [1] as its tool to stimulate the subcutaneous layer [2] by doing horizontal sweeping manipulation. Needling sites are mainly selected around or near tightened muscles (TM) that cause pain or other illnesses [3–5].

1.2 Tightened muscle (TM)

TMs are the muscles that are still in pathologically tense state when patients are relaxed under the condition that the central nervous system functions normally.

1.3 Pre-muscular diseases

Pre-muscular diseases refer to the diseases that cause chronic ischemia and oxygen deficit, leading to pathological tension of muscle and its subsidiary structure.

1.4 Real-muscular diseases

Real-muscular diseases are caused by pathological tension of the muscle and its subsidiary structure due to chronic ischemia and oxygen deficit.

1.5 Post-muscular diseases

Post-muscular diseases refer to a series of diseases caused by the muscles with pathological tensions that affects other organs (e.g., nerve or blood vessels) which are mostly distributed in or nearby the muscles.

1.6 Needle manipulation

Needle manipulation refers to pushing the needle to a proper depth after the needle is inserted into the subcutaneous layer.

1.7 Sweeping movement

Sweeping movement refers to a series of parallel and left-to-right movements of the needle in the subcutaneous layer after the needle manipulation.

1.8 Reperfusion approach

Reperfusion approach is to make tightened muscles contract vigorously within a short time and then relax in order to supply more blood to the ischemic part. It is suggested to provide equal force back by doctors when the muscles contract.

Reperfusion approach is often used during sweeping movement, and it can also be used separately for treatment of mild illnesses.

2. Basic characteristics of tightened muscle and its clinical evaluation

When patients relax their inspected area and their central nervous systems function normally, practitioners can still feel the "tightness, stiffness, hardness, and slipperiness" feelings when touching the targeting muscles with finger pulps. Patients often have spontaneous discomfort, pains, or obvious abnormal sensations. The joints that are associated with TMs are often weak and lack of strength. The range of joint activities is often reduced.

2.1 The clinical evaluation of tightened muscles

The muscle tension states are divided into five grades in clinical practice, which are defined as follows:

-: Muscles are soft and their activities are normal.

+: There is mild muscle tension without obvious clinical symptoms.

++: Muscles are moderately strained and stiff and are often accompanied by clinical symptoms which can often be reduced after a break.

+++: Muscles are tense and stiff with associated pains and other symptoms.

++++: Muscles are severely tense and stiff, and if touched with finger pulps, some changes like clumps and abnormal muscular band on the muscle belly can be felt. Severe intolerable painful symptoms are often accompanied. There is no relief after a break, and it even affects normal life.

2.2 Clinical manifestations of tightened muscles

Clinical manifestations of TMs can be divided into five major categories, including symptoms caused by TM directly or indirectly, by muscular internal organs, by dysfunctions of sleep, by emotions, and by those with unknown reasons.

2.2.1 The first major category

Clinical chief complaints that are directly caused by TMs: pain, dysfunction, and lack of power.

The main diseases include cervical spondylosis, tennis elbow, lumbar disc herniation, chronic knee pain, ankle sprain, etc.

The characteristics of muscle-induced pains:

a. Pains that are usually characterized by sourness, swelling, or tingling in rare cases.

b. Pain positioning is often inaccurate, and patients usually can only point out vague directions.

c. Peripheral muscle tissues or synergistic muscles are often affected.

d. Most of the pains can be relieved by hot compress and massage but not by pressure. Simple touching or rubbing the skin has no effect on the pain.

e. The degree of pain may aggravate when influenced by cool weather, muscle fatigue, lack of sleep, and bad mood.

f. Pain tends to decrease after using nonsteroidal analgesics, after the related muscles are relaxed, after the weather gets warmer, and after receiving massage and encountering emotional pleasure.

g. Long-term pain often causes changes in related bones and joints, such as hyperosteogeny, pseudospondylolisthesis, scoliosis, knee deformity, etc.

2.2.2 The second major category

TMs affect the internal or nearby nerves, arteries, and veins:

a. The main manifestations related to the affected nerves are the downstream symptoms of TMs, such as numbness.

b. The main manifestations related to the affected arteries are symptoms caused by TMs, such as headache, dizziness, chills, aversion to cold, contact temperature dropping, and even cold feeling of the whole body.

c. The main manifestations related to the affected veins are the downstream symptoms caused by TMs, such as edema, heaviness, itching, and skin darkening.

2.2.3 The third category

Pathological tension of neighboring skeletal muscles and muscular visceral lesions affects the body at the same time, and there is a close relationship between them; both of them often appear at the same time and disappear simultaneously after treatment. The clinical TM manifestations which belong to different systems of the human body are as follows:

a. Symptoms related to smooth muscles of the respiratory system include dry cough, chronic cough, asthma, chest short breath, breathing disorders, etc.

b. Symptoms related to heart muscle include chest tightness, palpitations, shortness of breath, chest pain, etc.

c. Symptoms related to gastrointestinal smooth muscles include stomach bloating, heartburn, acid regurgitation, belching, loss of appetite, emaciation, habitual constipation, chronic diarrhea, afraid of cold food cold drinks, etc.

d. Symptoms related to smooth muscles of the urinary system include urinary frequency, urgency, ureteral calculus, urine leakage, etc.

e. Symptoms related to smooth muscles of the reproductive and urinary system include:

i. Female: dysmenorrhea and menstrual abnormalities.

ii. Male: impotence, etc.

2.2.4 The fourth category

Symptoms related to mood and sleep, anxiety, insomnia, and mood swings.

2.2.5 The fifth category

A class of symptoms due to unknown causes, related to autonomic nervous dysfunctions and proprioceptive disorders.

Symptoms related to autonomic nervous dysfunction, such as abnormal sweating, continuous tears, continuous catarrhal rhinitis, excessive salivation, and discomfort of chest areas.

Symptoms related to proprioceptive disorders, such as imbalance, dizziness, tinnitus, weakness, and weight perception disorders.

2.3 How to check TMs

a. Mark the patient's painful positions.

b. List all possible muscles based on anatomical and biomechanical knowledge.

c. Use thumb pulp or pulps of index finger, middle finger, and ring finger to touch the muscular tensions of suspected muscles. If the muscular tension of one muscle is higher than its surrounding area, it can be diagnosed as pathological tight muscle.

3. Indications and contraindications

3.1 Indications

All indications of FSN are related to pathological tight muscles (**Figure 1**).

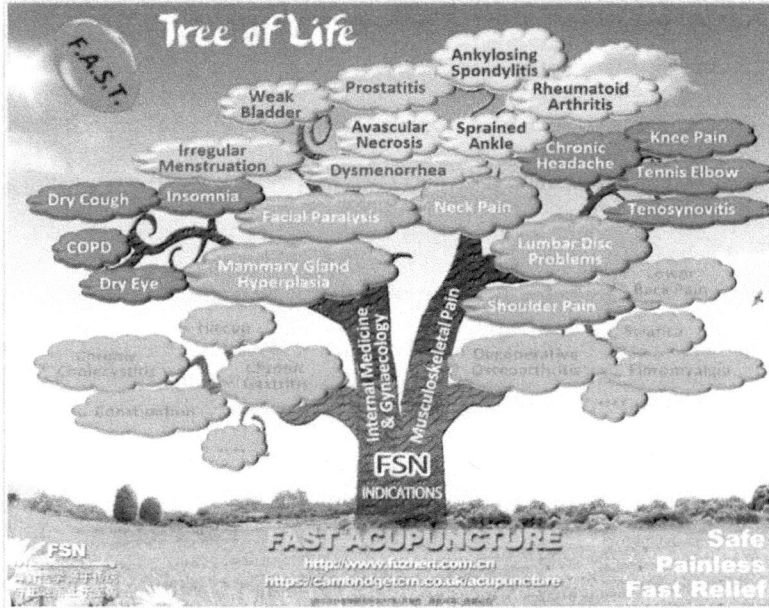

Figure 1.
The main indications.

3.1.1 Pre-muscular diseases

Ankylosing spondylitis, rheumatoid arthritis, asthma, gout, Parkinson's disease, facial paralysis, frozen shoulder, and so on.

3.1.2 Real-muscular diseases

Cervical spondylosis, tennis elbow, lumbar disc herniation, chronic knee pain, ankle sprain, headache, prostatitis, weak bladder (bladder leakage), hiccups, insomnia, depression, chronic cough, habitual constipation, and so on.

3.1.3 Post-muscular diseases

Dizziness, palpitation, chest tightness, local numbness, local edema, breast hyperplasia, cold disease, macular degeneration, diabetic foot, avascular necrosis of the femoral head, and so on.

3.2 Contraindications

- Patients with infectious diseases, malignant diseases, or patients with acute inflammation and fever.

- People with spontaneous bleeding or coagulopathy, which may result in nonstop bleeding after injury.

- Skin areas with infection, ulcer, scar, or tumor.

4. Operation steps and requirements

4.1 Determine the insertion point

The insertion points are chosen according to the following principles:

a. In most cases, insertion points are chosen nearby TM. It can be inserted 3–5 cm up, down, left, right, or oblique to the TM.

b. Insertion points are better to be nearby TMs for small area and less TMs, while insertion points are better to be far away for big area and more TMs.

c. From far to near, if there are several TMs, such as chronic cervical and lumbar pain, which is usually accompanied by abnormalities of the upper limbs and lower limbs, the insertion points should be chosen from far to near, rather than the opposite.

4.2 Needle selection and body position selection

4.2.1 Needle selection

The FSN inserting device and FSN acupuncture needle should be in accordance with the regulations of national medical device production and sales supervision. In order to prevent needling accidents, the disposable FSN acupuncture needle should be strictly inspected each time before use. If any unqualified conditions such as packaging damage are found, the needle should be eliminated.

4.2.1.1 FSN inserting device

FSN inserting device is a device specifically designed for the inserting of FSN acupuncture needle, which is developed by Nanjing FSN Medical Co., Ltd. It is convenient for the therapist to deliver the needle. It can not only reduce the pain of needle insertion but also ensure the accuracy and safety of the needling. The device consists of four parts, the base, the control button, the needle drive rod, and the groove, as shown in **Figure 2**.

4.2.1.2 FSN acupuncture needle

4.2.1.2.1 The structure of FSN acupuncture needle

The FSN acupuncture needle consists of three components. The combination of the three components is shown in **Figure 3**.

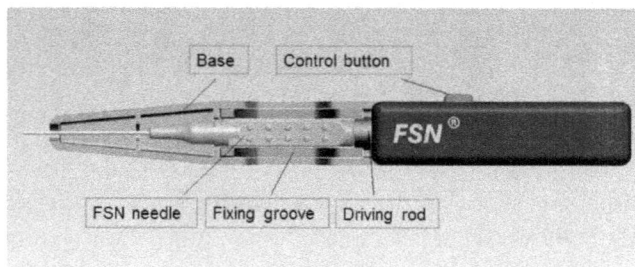

Figure 2.
FSN acupuncture needle in the FSN inserting device.

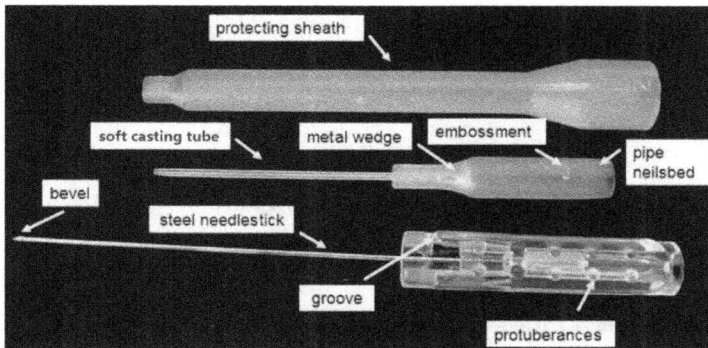

Figure 3.
The three parts of FSN acupuncture needle.

4.2.1.2.2 FSN acupuncture needle core

The needle core consists of a stainless steel needle and a hard-plastic core, as shown in **Figure 2**. This part insures the FSN acupuncture needle to reach enough rigidity to enter the body quickly and to complete sweeping movement. The stainless steel needle tip is beveled. On the base, there are 10 protuberances which are on one side. When the convex protuberances are upward, the beveled tip of the needle is also upward. The surface is in line with the tip of the needle, the front end of the needle has a longitudinal groove, and the front of the groove has a transverse slot on the right side, which is used for fixing the soft casting tube during performing a sweeping movement.

4.2.1.2.3 Soft casting tube and base of FSN acupuncture needle

The soft casting tube covers the stainless steel needle (steel needle inside, soft casting tube outside). The soft casting tube is fixed to the plastic socket through the built-in rivets, as shown in **Figure 2**. The casting tube of FSN acupuncture needle has a bump, which is matched with the grooves in the core seat and the slot. The protuberances on the base are placed at the bottom of the groove when we sweep the needle.

The main function of the soft casting tube:

a. The tube and the core are anastomosed into one, which is conductive to the stability of the insertion, as well as to the needle manipulation and the sweeping movement.

b. When performing sweeping movement, the stainless steel needle tip is fully retreated into the soft tube; it can prevent the tingling caused by injuring the blood vessels.

c. Because of its sufficient softness, the tube which will not affect normal activities of patients can be kept under the skin for several hours after the treatment, and it will not puncture blood vessels and other tissues.

4.2.1.2.4 Protective sheath

To protect the stainless steel needle and soft tube from the impact of the collision, we designed a protective sheath. The protective sheath is used to protect the aseptic state, as shown in **Figure 2**. After the sweeping movement, the solid needle should not be discarded. It must be put back into the protective sheath to prevent puncturing oneself and others.

4.2.1.2.5 Length, diameter, appearance, and preservation of FSN acupuncture needle

4.2.1.2.6 Appearance of FSN acupuncture needle

FSN acupuncture needle is disposable and can only be used for one time; it is also known as disposable subcutaneous acupuncture needle with plastic tube, as shown in **Figure 2** and **Table 1**.

4.2.1.2.7 Use and storage of FSN acupuncture needles

The FSN acupuncture needle is a presterilized product for disposable use. Please do not use once the package is damaged. After opening the package, you must make sure that the surface of the needle is bright and clean, the needle is not rough and defective, the casting tube is transparent, and the needle is sharp. If any problem is found, please stop using it and notify the manufacturer immediately.

The FSN acupuncture needle should be kept in a dry, cool area.

4.2.2 Body position

Common body positions are as follows:

a. Supine position: Mainly suitable for the insertion points of the head, chest, abdomen, and upper and lower extremities.

b. Lateral position: Mainly suitable for insertion points on either side and upper and lower extremities of the body.

c. Prone position: Mainly suitable for the insertion points on the head, back, hip, and lower extremities. A pillow is placed under the patient's chest; the patient's hands are folded on the forehead.

d. Orthopnea position: Mainly suitable for the insertion points of the neck, shoulder, upper back and upper extremities, the knees, and the lower extremity regions.

e. Sitting with head down position: Suitable for the insertion points of the occipital and upper neck regions.

4.3 Disinfection and needle insertion

4.3.1 Disinfection

Sterilize the local skin: Routine skin disinfection.

	Solid needle(mm)	Soft tube (mm)
Length	52	49
Diameter	0.6	1.05

Table 1.
The size of the FSN acupuncture needle.

Sterilize the upper part of FSN inserting device: Use alcoholic cotton to clean the upper part of FSN inserting device.

4.3.2 Needle insertion

After removing the plastic protection tube, place the needle into the inserting device; make sure the side with protuberance (with dots) is facing upward, and then pull the groove back to the load situation. Hold the device with middle finger at the bottom of the device, index finger on the red trigger button, and thumb on the top, as shown in **Figure 4**.

Place the upper part of FSN inserting device on the disinfected skin of inserting point; the angle between the device and the skin should be as small as possible. With the cooperation of the left hand, the operator presses the trigger button, and then the needle penetrates quickly into the subcutaneous layer as shown in **Figure 5**.

With the left index finger and thumb holding the needle, pull the needle out of the groove, and then the right hand withdraws the inserting device as shown in **Figure 6**.

4.4 Manipulation and sweeping

4.4.1 Manipulation

After inserting the needle, if the needle is directly inserted into the muscle, the patient will feel soreness, and the practitioner's hand that is holding the needle may also feel the resistance at the same time. In this case, the practitioner should pull the needle handle with the thumb, index finger, and middle finger slowly backward out of the muscle layer and back to the subcutaneous layer.

After confirming the needle tip is inside the subcutaneous layer, the practitioner can put down the needle body, and then prepare for the manipulation. During which, the practitioner holds the needle with the right hand and pushes the needle forward along the subcutaneous layer. It is better to raise the needle tip slightly up when pushing so that the tip is slightly tilted, making sure the needle does not penetrate into the muscle layer. When the needle is being pushed forward, the skin is lined up. During the process, if the patient feels sudden tingling or the practitioner feels sudden resistance, it is usually because the needle tip penetrates the blood vessel wall. Therefore, the needle manipulation process should be as slow as possible. When the practitioner feels the resistance before the patient feels pains, it is better to quickly withdraw the needle slightly, and then adjust the needle direction upward or downward to avoid causing pains to the patient.

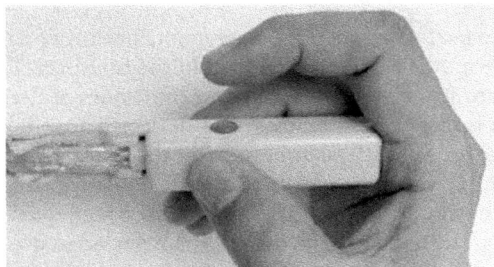

Figure 4.
Gesture for holding inserting device.

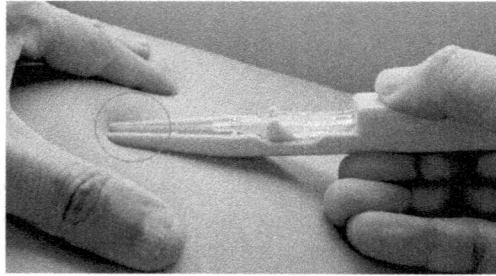

Figure 5.
Before inserting the needle, the positional relationship between the inserting device and the skin.

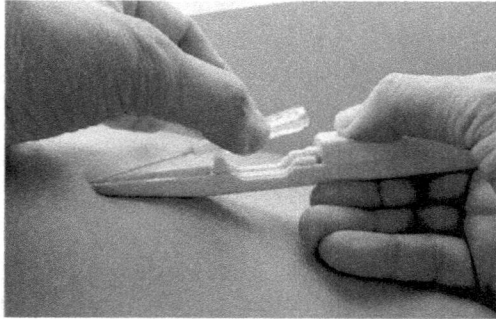

Figure 6.
After inserting, the right hand is fixed, and the left hand pinches the needle.

Generally, it is suggested to go as deep as all soft tube being under the skin. In some other cases, if the needle is inserted near the side of the finger joint or other facet joints, the soft tube need not be fully embedded subcutaneously.

4.4.2 Sweeping movement

4.4.2.1 Manipulation

When the needle is in the correct position, with the left hand fixing the soft tube seat, the practitioner can use the right hand to recede the core needle and fix the protuberance of the soft tube seat in the slot of the core seat. At this time, the needle tip is no longer exposed outside but has returned to the soft tube, almost in line with the soft tube.

Then it is ready to perform sweeping movement. The inner nail margin of the right thumb and the middle finger is used to hold the core base, the index finger and the ring finger are separated on the left and right sides of the middle finger, and the tip of the thumb is fixed on the skin as the fulcrum. The index finger and the ring finger sweep in a seesaw-like sector one after the other. The scope of sweeping movements is better to be as large as possible, with stable speed and enough power, and sweeping rhythm should be slow so as to avoid the feeling of numbness, swelling, and pain. During the sweeping process, it is suggested to use the right hand to operate, while the left hand cooperates with reperfusion approach (**Figure 7**).

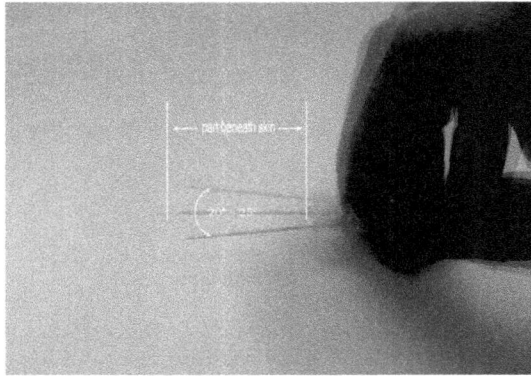

Figure 7.
The swaying movement.

4.4.2.2 Types of sweeping movement

According to different ways of swinging the needle, the sweeping movement is divided into the following two categories:

a. Horizontal sweeping movement: The sweeping action of the needle tip is at the same horizontal level, which can save strength and is used more often. It can be used in most cases. Right now, with the cooperation of reperfusion approach, horizontal sweeping is mostly used during clinical practice.

b. Sweeping movement in an elliptical circle: The solid needle moves clockwise or counterclockwise under the skin to perform a circular or oval movement, applicable for intractable diseases (see **Figure 8**).

4.4.2.3 Time and frequency of sweeping movement

Each needling point can be swept for 2 minutes with a frequency of 200 times per minute. Practitioner can check and assess muscle tension after 30 seconds of sweeping.

4.5 Reperfusion approach

During the FSN manipulation, reperfusion approach targeting PTMs is accompanied.

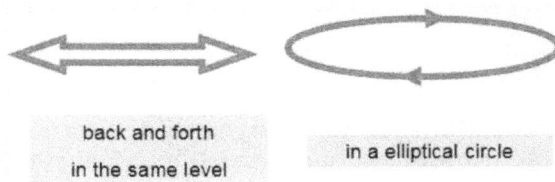

Figure 8.
Types of sweeping movement.

4.5.1 Classification of reperfusion

Active reperfusion refers to a reperfusion approach that is completed by the patient without assistance.

Passive reperfusion refers to a reperfusion approach that is completed by patients through reliance on external efforts.

4.5.2 Operational requirements of reperfusion approach

4.5.2.1 Range (as wide as possible)

According to the anatomy of the muscle and its functional activity, the practitioner should guide the patient to achieve maximum radius of the muscle (isotonic contraction) or maximum intensity of the muscle (equal length contraction).

4.5.2.2 Slow speed

A pause of 1–3 seconds is required during the maximum radius and the maximum intensity and relaxation. It is recommended to complete a reperfusion approach at around 10 seconds.

4.5.2.3 Less number of times

The same group of reperfusion approach, which refers to activity at the same direction and the same angle, should not be repeated more than three times.

4.5.2.4 Length of interval

A half hour interval is required between two groups of reperfusion activities so that the muscles could get enough relaxation.

4.5.2.5 Changes

Some targeted changes could be made in the reperfusion approach for intractable pains.

4.5.3 Operating methods of reperfusion approach

Reperfusion approach is different in different parts of the body. During clinical practice, Reperfusion approach should be designed according to joint features and the distribution of TMs related to targeted diseases:

a. Neck: Six main movements are recommended, including lowering head, raising head, turning head to the left or right side, revolving head, and so on.

b. Shoulder: Combing hair, trying to reach scapula of the same side, raising arms, and so on.

c. Waist: Holding head with hands and bowing forward on the treatment couch, flying fish posture, twisting butt from left to right, stepping movement on the same position, voluntary cough, and so on.

d. Knee: Flexion and extension, stepping movement on the same position.

e. Chest, back: Taking deep breath, voluntary cough.

4.6 Retaining and removing of the soft tube

When the sweeping movement is finished, the solid needle can be taken out and placed into the protective sleeve. Put a piece of adhesive tape to cover the tube seat, and fix it on the skin. Make sure that the adhesive tape can cover the entire soft tube so that the soft tube kept under the skin can be fixed.

4.6.1 Time length for retaining the soft tube

It is usually suggested to retain the soft tube for 1 hour, and the retaining time can vary according to different clinical situations. Doctors can decide the retaining time by taking into consideration factors like weather conditions, patient's reaction, and severity of disease. If the weather is hot, the patient sweats easily, or the patient has itching feeling around the needling point or surrounding area due to allergic reaction to the adhesive tape; the retaining time is better not to be long; otherwise, the retaining time can be longer.

4.6.2 Remove the soft tube

To remove the soft tube, use the left thumb and index finger to fix surrounding skin of the needling point, then hold the soft tube seat with the right thumb and index finger, and take it out gently and slowly. Use a sterile cotton ball to press the needling point so as to prevent bleeding. After removal of the soft tube, patients can leave after a short break.

4.7 Time intervals and treatment course

4.7.1 Time intervals

Chronic diseases can be treated on a daily basis for two–three continuous treatment, and then the time interval can be prolonged to 2 to 3 days between two treatments. For other problems, the time interval can be decided according to the treatment effect.

4.7.2 Treatment course

Three times of treatment are usually considered as a course of treatment.

5. Exception and its handling

5.1 Subcutaneous bruises

A small amount of subcutaneous bleeding and local small pieces of bruising will disappear and recover automatically; generally no special treatment is needed. But practitioners need to explain to the patient so as to eliminate the patient's worries and fears.

If the local swelling and pain are obvious or the bruised area is large and affects functional activities, practitioners need to withdraw the needle immediately and apply cold compresses to stop bleeding. After 24 hours, hot compress and mild massage can be applied to promote the dissipation of blood stasis.

5.2 Fainting during the treatment

5.2.1 Prevention of fainting during treatment

It is better to explain thoroughly to the patient so as to eliminate the patient's worries, choose the right position, and treat the patient in a gentle way. If the patient feels hungry and tired, treatment can be given after the patient finishes eating, drinking, and taking a rest. Supine position is recommended when patients feel too nervous. Practitioners should observe the patients' responses and ask about their feelings. If the treatment causes discomfort and the patient shows symptoms of fainting, the practitioner should stop immediately and take some necessary measures in advance.

5.2.2 Management of fainting during treatment

The needling operation should be stopped immediately. The practitioner should withdraw the needle, help the patients lie on bed, and keep them warm. Generally, the patient will recover soon after drinking warm water or sugar water and taking some rest. If the patient is still unconscious or breathing weakly, or his or her blood pressure drops rapidly, other rescuing measures or first aid treatment should be carried out.

6. Precautions

- It is suggested to give a brief explanation to patients about FSN manipulation and its features before giving treatment so as to reduce the patient's fear and doubts.

- For patients who are aged and weak, the first time to receive FSN treatment and patients who are scared of needles, it is suggested to treat them by supine position.

- When giving reperfusion approach, the scope of activity should be from small to large, step by step, and the external force given from outside should be from light to heavy. The external force should be counterforce when patients move actively. A sudden force or vigorous activity is forbidden when giving passive activity. Age, physical, mental state, and other factors of patients should be considered when practitioners design the reperfusion activities. It is better to avoid the situation that one single reperfusion approach takes too much time, too much strength, or is repeated too frequently.

- During the period of retaining the soft tube, patients should keep adhesive tape clean and dry so as to avoid infections. Mild activities are suggested during the retaining of the soft tube, but strong and large movements should be avoided in order not to affect the fixation of the soft tube. In some rare cases, if the retaining tube reaches the blood vessels, resulting in stinging or bleeding, the tube should be taken out immediately. Do not be worried if patients feel itchy around the tube-retaining area, as it is usually due to allergic reactions of patients to the soft tube or adhesive tape. Practitioners can choose other kinds of materials instead to fix the tube, for example, bandages can be used.

- Practitioners should not perform FSN therapy on the abdomen of women within 3 months of pregnancy. Even for women who are pregnant over

3 months, it is better not to conduct needling on the lumbosacral region and abdomen. If pregnant women are nervous, it is forbidden to do needling treatment.

- If patients use safflower oil, massage milk, and other stimulating drugs for external use on their skin or receive treatment of strong plaster, strong cupping, and scraping method, FSN therapy should not be applied in a short time. But if the skin condition has returned to normal after these treatments, then it is suitable to do FSN therapy.

- It is better not to give FSN therapy to people who have recently received steroids injection therapy.

Author details

Zhonghua Fu[1*] and Dejian Lu[2]

1 Nanjing FSN Medical Institute, Nanjing, China

2 Department of Traditional Chinese Medicine, Kiang Wu Hospital, Macau, China

*Address all correspondence to: 139004426@qq.com

IntechOpen

References

[1] Fu ZH. The Foundation of Fu's Subcutaneous Needling. Beijing: People's Medical Publishing House; 2016

[2] Fu ZH, Wang JH, Sun JH, Chen XY, Xu JG. Fu's subcutaneous needling: Possible clinical evidence of the subcutaneous connective tissue in acupuncture. Journal of Alternative and Complementary Medicine. 2007;**13**(1):47-52

[3] Fu ZH. The Manual of Fu's Subcutaneous Needling for Painful Problems. Beijing: People's Medical Publishing House; 2011

[4] FU Z-h, CHEN X-y, LU L-j, LIN J, XU J-g. Immediate effect of Fu's subcutaneous needling for low back pain. Chinese Medical Journal. 2006;**119**(11):953-956

[5] Fu Z, Hsieh Y-L, Hong C-Z, Kao M-J, Lin J-G, Chou L-W. Remote subcutaneous needling to suppress the irritability of Myofascial trigger spots: An experimental study in rabbits. Evidence-based Complementary and Alternative Medicine. 2012;**2012**:353916

Scalp Acupuncture and Mental Disorders

Chuen Heung Yau and Cheuk Long Ip

Abstract

While conventional treatments for many mental problems remain problematic and unsatisfactory in therapeutic outcomes, there is great demand for an effective yet economical treatment method that can alleviate the suffering of psychiatric patients. In traditional Chinese medicine, acupuncture on the scalp has been used for centuries. Not until recent decades did acupuncturists and clinicians develop new understandings and theories on the effect of scalp acupuncture. Upon elaboration on the therapeutic value of scalp acupuncture, it shows great potential in treating mental health disorders including depression, anxiety disorders, schizophrenia, and insomnia. Its profound treatment outcome in clinical use has caught clinicians' attention in recent years. However, controlled studies and investigations on its effect on psychiatric problems remain relatively small in number, and determinative evidence has yet to be found. In order to provide conclusive evidence on the use of scalp acupuncture to these disorders, more data from high-quality controlled trials are urgently needed. Since scalp acupuncture has advantages over the use of traditional acupuncture or body acupuncture in clinical and investigation settings, we are expecting a shift of attention from individualized acupuncture to a standardized universal scalp acupuncture treatment in clinical practice and academia.

Keywords: scalp acupuncture, treatment, mental disorder

1. Introduction

Mental disorders have been one of the leading contributors to the global disease burden in the twenty-first century. It has been accounted for one-third of the global disability [1]. Owing to the absence of cost-effective interventions and preventive measures, the prevalence of mental disorders shows no sign of declination. Surveys have shown that the increase in rates of treatments and therefore an even larger demand for mental health services has become an evitable problem for the society [2]. A proportion of patients with mental health problems shift from conventional health service to complementary and alternative medicine (CAM) [3]. Various studies showed the 12-month prevalence of CAM ranging from 10 to 75%, depending on populations and research methods [4]. Among all CAM applicable to patients, acupuncture, as one of the components in traditional Chinese medicine (TCM), has been commonly used in East Asian countries including China and Taiwan [5, 6]. In contrast to traditional body acupuncture, treatments for mental illness are more focused on acupuncture on the scalp. The sole use of acupoints or lines on the scalp in acupuncture deviates from the concept of traditional acupuncture and named scalp acupuncture. The development of scalp acupuncture has been rapid in the recent decades, and there is emerging evidence in supporting its use in patients with mental illnesses.

2. History of scalp acupuncture

The earliest medical record for the application of acupuncture on scalps can be traced back to around 5 BC [7]. Since then, experiences accumulated with the utilization of acupuncture on the scalp in treating various illnesses. Along with the establishment of TCM theories, it had been a component in traditional acupuncture system. Until the 1950s, acupuncture experts started to observe and recognize the relationship between illnesses and subscalp spots. Inspired by micropuncture systems concepts and influenced by anatomical and physiological knowledge from modern medicine, new theories and new needling techniques had been established [8]. In the 1970s, acupuncturists from different areas of China developed their own schools of theory, and several scalp acupuncture systems have been suggested. Despite variations present in theoretical concepts, sites of acupuncture (acupoints), and nomenclature among different schools, many areas such as the clinical indication and treatment procedures share common ground. Most recognized theories include the adaptation of knowledge in cerebral anatomy, physiology, neurology, and reflexology. Owing to the impressive therapeutic effect of scalp acupuncture in treating brain diseases as well as other illnesses, there was a strong urge to facilitate academic exchange and promote scalp acupuncture to wider communities. Intensive efforts had been made in standardizing the names of the scalp acupoints. By the time the World Health Organization (WHO) set up an international standard scalp acupuncture nomenclature systems in 1989, scalp acupuncture had been already extensively applied by therapists and acupuncturists around the globe [9]. Some places like the USA and Japan had even developed their own understandings in the field of scalp acupuncture [10, 11]. In short, scalp acupuncture is a technique derived from TCM, yet its theory and application involves multiplicity of systems that have been rapidly developing in the recent decades.

3. Modern adaptation of scalp acupuncture in mental disorders

In TCM concepts, all patients can be categorized into different syndrome types despite the diagnosis of disease. Patients will then be prescribed with a unique treatment regimen, i.e., two patients suffering from the same disease might receive prescription of different acupoints since they may vary in syndrome type [12]. This individualized medicine concept has been a feature of TCM since the early establishment of the philosophy of TCM. However, there are few shortcomings for this manipulation. Firstly, the differentiation of syndrome types may not be accurate or definite as the diagnosis procedures are highly dependent to the therapists' clinical experience. Besides, since most patients with mental problems have complicated somatic problems or being masked by the side effects of psychiatric medication, diagnosis of syndrome type according to TCM theories may become exceptionally difficult. Moreover, individualized acupuncture treatment may provide inconsistent therapeutic outcomes. Objective observation and comparisons of the treatment results become impossible as the testing subjects are using different acupoints. As a result, we suggest the use of standardized, identical acupoint regimen for acupuncture treatment on psychiatric patients.

Instead of body acupuncture, scalp acupuncture has been widely used in diseases originated from the brain. The invention of scalp acupuncture has been with accordance to the neurology and reflexology knowledge of the brain and scalp structures. It is perceived that acupuncture stimulation on the subscalpular tissue may exert influences to the respective lesion in the brain [7]. A large proportion of preceding clinical trials of acupuncture on various mental illnesses such as anxiety, depression, and insomnia adopted the essential use of scalp acupuncture, while the collateral use of body acupuncture remains elective [13–15]. The sole use of scalp acupuncture in treating insomnia or other diseases such as intracerebral hemorrhage and Parkinson's disease has been endorsed in literatures [15–17]. Therefore, we are convinced that the use of scalp acupuncture will be sufficient to bring about therapeutic value to the psychiatric patients.

Besides, scalp acupuncture shows superiority over body acupuncture in clinical situations. Unlike body acupuncture, patients receiving scalp acupuncture are not required to retain on bed. They can sit on chairs or carry out static activities during treatment sessions. Another advantage of scalp acupuncture is that since textile sensitivity of the scalp is relatively low, scalp acupuncture would cause less pain and discomfort when compared with body acupuncture. Apart from diminished unpleasant sensation during needle insertion, the manipulation of scalp acupuncture cannot be easily seen by the treatment recipients. This is important especially to those patients who easily feel anxious upon seeing needles.

4. Procedures of scalp acupuncture

In practice of scalp acupuncture, sterile disposable acupuncture needles of the standard size of 0.20 × 25 mm or 0.22 × 25 mm are usually used. Acupuncture needles are obliquely inserted onto the selected acupoints with an angle of 15–30° after standard sterilization procedures. The needles should be inserted at a depth of 10 mm lying between aponeurosis layer and loose areolar connective tissue. Needles rest too deep or too shadow at the scalp structure will cause pain and diminished effect. After the insertion, mild stimulation to the needles is recommended. Needles can be swirled at time intervals. A standard session of scalp acupuncture treatment will last for at least an hour before the needles are carefully removed after the treatment.

5. Selection of acupoints in treating mental disorders

According to TCM theories, acupoints are explicit points located at the surface of our bodies. Each acupoint serves its own function and can be joined together to form meridian lines. The selection and combination of acupoints is the most crucial component in acupuncture therapy. For example, it is understandable that the use of acupoints in treating brain diseases is definitely distinct from those for alleviating pain problems such as back pains. In the treatment of mental problems or brain organic problems, acupoints and scalp lines on the scalp including Baihui, Sishencong, midline of the forehead, lateral line 2 of the forehead and posterior lateral Line of the Vertex are commonly used.

Baihui is located at the vertex of the midline of the head, which is the meeting point from apexes of ears. It is one of the acupoints on the governor vessel (GV). The governor vessel is known to have its passage running from the coccyx upward along the spine into the brain. Under the TCM theory, it is the convergence of all Yang meridians and thus stimulation at Baihui can boost the flow of Qi in all the

Yang meridians, benefits brain development, and enhances intelligence. In modern studies, Baihui has been comprehensively studied and applied in treating a variety of brain diseases and mood disorders such as intracerebral hemorrhage, dementia, depression, anxiety, insomnia, etc. [13, 18–20].

Around the site Baihui locates the acupoints Sishencong. Sishencong is the four points located at 1 cun anterior, posterior, and lateral to Baihui. They are excluded from the 12 main meridians. Sishencong is known for its calming effect as well as tranquilizing excitement in mood. Different directions of needle insertion at Sishencong, such as pointing toward or away from Baihui or toward the side of brain lesion, can bring about different therapeutic effects. In general, it facilitates the harmony of Yin and Yang.

The location of the midline of forehead, also known as Shenting is 0.5 cun above the hairline and within the midline. Similar to Sishencong, it has been used to calm emotions and improve poor memory in theory. Lateral line 2 of the forehead are two acupoints located 0.5 cun above the hairline and directly above the pupils. In reference to anatomy, the midline and lateral line 2 of the forehand are the site of the prefrontal cortex (PFC). There are mainly five functions of PFC, which are executive functions, memory, intelligence, language, and gaze control. Because of the rich cortical and subcortical connection, PFC can initiate and perform goal-directed patterns of behavior, short-term memory tasks, planning, problem solving, etc. [21].

Posterior lateral lines of vertex are two points that are 1 cun next to the posterior Sishencong. It is located at posterior parietal lobe, anterior to the occipital lobe, and posterior to primary somatosensory cortex. Together with the close interconnection with frontal premotor area, it serves as a sensory-motor interface [22]. It receives sensory input from somatosensory cortex, and other regions of the brain integrate the information to allow the executive functioning.

6. Mechanism of scalp acupuncture

Acupuncture for treating brain diseases is never mythical or ritual. It has originated from years of clinical experience and scientific proofs. Scalp acupuncture has proven to bring both functional and structural changes to the brain. Study has shown that scalp acupuncture at Sishencong can significantly decrease the heart rate and blood pressure of the test subjects. It is suggested that it exerts its effect through modulation of autonomic nervous system [23]. Another physiological change induced by scalp acupuncture is the regulation of perfusion in the brain. An alteration of perfusion among brain structures is detected under the inspection of single-photon emission computerized tomography (SPECT) [7, 24]. It is suggested to be the action of vasoconstrictor endothelin-1 (ET-1) [25]. The dysfunction of the brain structures in brain diseases and injuries can be detected and depicted by the probe of abnormal brainwaves [26]. Scalp acupuncture has shown its ability in restoring normal waveforms in healthy and depressed patients [27, 28]. In the long term, acupuncture provokes modulation at cortical structures including orbitofrontal cortex and prefrontal cortex and medial temporal lobes, together with limbic regions of hypothalamus, amygdala, cingulate, and hippocampus. The effects of acupuncture on these structures have been strongly supported by neuroimaging data obtained from electroencephalography (EEG), fMRI, magnetoencephalography (MEG), and positron emission tomography (PET) [29].

Altered catecholamine levels are commonly found in patients with mental illness. The use of scalp acupuncture has been suggest to bring about a surge of neurohormones and neurotransmitters in the central nervous system such as adrenocorticotropic hormone (ACTH), beta-endorphins, γ-aminobutyric acid (GABA) protein, noradrenaline, and serotonin [30, 31]. Other molecules such as brain-derived neurotrophic factor (BDNF), postsynaptic density-95 (PSD-95) protein, and nitric oxide synthase (NOS) also respond to scalp acupuncture, suggesting their possible participation to the mechanism of action [32, 33].

7. Indication for scalp acupuncture on mental disorders

There has been a long history of utilizing acupuncture in treating mental health problems and "mind-related" syndromes in ancient China. However, scientific literatures and clinical trials on acupuncture for mental problems had not been recorded until 1980s. Despite numerous clinical observations and controlled trials that have been made since then, evidences have remain insufficient to draw a definitive conclusion on the general use of acupuncture on psychiatric patients. More high-quality controlled trials with greater sample size and longer follow-up period are clearly needed in order to advocate the use of scalp acupuncture for treating mental illness.

7.1 Depression

Depression is the most common mental problem [34]. The disappointing response rate and side effects of conventional medication discourage a proportion of patients from complying conventional treatments. Instead, they turn to CAM treatments, including scalp acupuncture. Meta-analysis has shown possible efficacy of scalp acupuncture on major depressive and bipolar disorders and antepartum and post-stroke depressions [14, 35]. Several studies suggested that the effect of scalp acupuncture is comparable to conventional medication, while a study concluded better outcome in somatization and cognitive process disturbances over antidepressant [36]. Despite various clinical investigations that have been carried out, additional high-quality randomized controlled trials are urgently needed to provide conclusive evidence [37].

7.2 Anxiety disorders

Controlled studies have obtained consistent positive results on the use of acupuncture in patients suffering from anxiety disorder. However, most investigations have been focused on preoperative anxiety, generalized anxiety disorder, or anxiety neurosis only, while there is a large vacancy of knowledge about the effect of acupuncture on specific anxiety disorders like panic disorder, phobias, or obsessive-compulsive disorders [13]. A recent meta-analysis advocates the use of acupuncture on patients having post-traumatic stress disorder (PTSD) [38]. It is worth mentioning that a large proportion of studies concerning anxiety have been utilizing auricular acupuncture and body acupuncture, whereas investigations on the use of scalp acupuncture are scarce. We can see a great demand for complementing our knowledge toward the use of scalp acupuncture on various anxiety disorders.

7.3 Schizophrenia and psychotic disorders

Relatively few studies have been made on the use of scalp acupuncture to psychotic patients. Most studies suggested limited evidence on the use of acupuncture as adjuvant treatment along with antipsychotic medication. However, a general significant improvement in sleep quality and extrapyramidal side effects has been observed in psychotic patients receiving acupuncture treatment [35, 39].

7.4 Insomnia

Insomnia and sleep disorders are common mental health problems that have been always overlooked. Poor sleep quality could adversely affect the quality of life and deteriorate mental status. The use of acupuncture and scalp acupuncture may benefit insomnia patients, according to recent systematic review literatures. Since the current results of the clinical studies are promising and consistent, the use of acupuncture may be encouraged as an adjunctive therapy in insomnia [15]. We are expecting more high-quality evidence supporting especially the use of scalp acupuncture in the treatment of insomnia in the near future.

8. Contraindication of scalp acupuncture

The contraindications of scalp acupuncture include infants with unclosed cranial fontanelles and sutures. Patients with cranial infection, ulcer, or scars on scalp are not advised to perform scalp acupuncture. Patients with past history of epilepsy or seizure should be comprehensively evaluated by the therapists before receiving treatment. Patients extremely anxious toward needles should be handled with care. Appropriate counseling and encouragement will be useful in building a good rapport between therapist and the parent. Possible side effect of scalp acupuncture includes discomfort or mild pain by the needle, emotional distress during the treatment sessions, bleeding, sleep disturbance, and increased hyperactivity.

9. Summary

Scalp acupuncture deserves greater concerns on its application on mental disorders. It has advantages over conventional individualized body acupuncture in clinical practice, and its effect could be objectively observed. Evidence from neuro-imaging, biochemical investigations, and clinical trial has been supporting the use of scalp acupuncture on patients with mental disorders. We see great potential in scalp acupuncture to play an important role in alleviating or even preventing mental health problems in the future. Nonetheless, there is an urgent need for quality trials to provide definitive evidence to support the use of scalp acupuncture for various mental disorders.

List of abbreviations

CAM	complementary and alternative medicine
ET-1	endothelin-1
EEG	electroencephalography
fMRI	functional magnetic resonance imaging
GABA	γ-aminobutyric acid
GV	governor vessel
MEG	magnetoencephalography
MRI	magnetic resonance imaging
NOS	nitric oxide synthase
PET	positron emission tomography
PTSD	post-traumatic stress disorder
PFC	prefrontal cortex

PSD-95	postsynaptic density-95 protein
SPECT	single-photon emission computerized tomography
TCM	traditional Chinese medicine
WHO	World Health Organization

Author details

Chuen Heung Yau* and Cheuk Long Ip
School of Chinese Medicine, Hong Kong Baptist University, Hong Kong

*Address all correspondence to: annyau@hkbu.edu.hk

IntechOpen

References

[1] Vigo D, Thornicroft G, Atun R. Estimating the true global burden of mental illness. The Lancet Psychiatry. 2016;**3**(2):171-178

[2] Jorm AF, Patten SB, Brugha TS, Mojtabai R. Has increased provision of treatment reduced the prevalence of common mental disorders? Review of the evidence from four countries. World Psychiatry. 2017;**16**(1):90-99

[3] Kessler RC, Demler O, Frank RG, Olfson M, Pincus HA, Walters EE, et al. Prevalence and treatment of mental disorders, 1990 to 2003. The New England Journal of Medicine. 2005;**352**(24):2515-2523

[4] Gureje O, Nortje G, Makanjuola V, Oladeji BD, Seedat S, Jenkins R. The role of global traditional and complementary systems of medicine in the treatment of mental health disorders. The Lancet Psychiatry. 2015;**2**(2):168-177

[5] Thirthalli J, Zhou L, Kumar K, Gao J, Vaid H, Liu H, et al. Traditional, complementary, and alternative medicine approaches to mental health care and psychological wellbeing in India and China. The Lancet Psychiatry. 2016;**3**(7):660-672

[6] Hsu MC, Creedy D, Moyle W, Venturato L, Tsay SL, Ouyang WC. Use of complementary and alternative medicine among adult patients for depression in Taiwan. Journal of Affective Disorders. 2008;**111**(2-3):360-365

[7] Liu Z, Guan L, Wang Y, Xie CL, Lin XM, Zheng GQ. History and mechanism for treatment of intracerebral hemorrhage with scalp acupuncture. Evidence-based Complementary and Alternative Medicine. 2012;**2012**:895032

[8] Jiao SF. Scalp Acupuncture. Taiyuan, China: Shanxi People's Publishing House; 1982

[9] World Health Organization. A proposed standard international acupuncture nomenclature: Report of a WHO scientific group. Geneva: World Health Organization; 1991

[10] Yamamoto T. New scalp acupuncture. Acupuncture in Medicine. 1989;**6**(2):46-48

[11] Zhu M. Zhu's Scalp Acupuncture. San Francisco, Calif.: 8 Dragons Publishing; 1992

[12] Guo RJ, Wang JL, Zhang YL. Analysis on the relevance of elements of TCM syndromes in depression patients. Journal of Traditional Chinese Medicine. 2008;**9**:035

[13] Pilkington K. Anxiety, depression and acupuncture: A review of the clinical research. Autonomic Neuroscience. 2010;**157**(1-2):91-95

[14] Zhang ZJ, Chen HY, Yip KC, Ng R, Wong VT. The effectiveness and safety of acupuncture therapy in depressive disorders: Systematic review and meta-analysis. Journal of Affective Disorders. 2010;**124**(1-2):9-21

[15] Ryu CG, Kim SJ, Cho AR, Seo JH, Jeong SS, Lee JS, et al. A review of scalp acupuncture on patients with insomnia-focusing on Chinese journals. Journal of Oriental Neuropsychiatry. 2012;**23**(1):17-29

[16] Zheng GQ , Zhao ZM, Wang Y, Gu Y, Li Y, Chen XM, et al. Meta-analysis of scalp acupuncture for acute hypertensive intracerebral hemorrhage. The Journal of Alternative and Complementary Medicine. 2011;**17**(4):293-299

[17] Lee HS, Park HL, Lee SJ, Shin BC, Choi JY, Lee MS. Scalp acupuncture for Parkinson's disease: A systematic review of randomized controlled trials.

Chinese Journal of Integrative Medicine. 2013;**19**(4):297-306

[18] Wang WW, Xie CL, Lu L, Zheng GQ. A systematic review and meta-analysis of Baihui (GV20)-based scalp acupuncture in experimental ischemic stroke. Scientific Reports. 2014;**4**:3981

[19] Xin-sheng L, Yong H. Comparative study on the effect of Baihui (GV 20), Shuigou (GV 26) and Shenmen (HT 7) on cognition of patients with vascular dementia. Journal of Acupuncture and Tuina Science. 2005;**3**(5):20-23

[20] Yeung WF, Chung KF, Zhang SP, Yap TG, Law AC. Electroacupuncture for primary insomnia: A randomized controlled trial. Sleep. 2009;**32**(8):1039-1047

[21] Luria AR. Higher Cortical Functions in Man. New York: Springer Science & Business Media; 2012

[22] Matelli M, Luppino G. Parietofrontal circuits for action and space perception in the macaque monkey. NeuroImage. 2001;**14**(1):S27-S32

[23] Hsu CC, Weng CS, Sun MF, Shyu LY, Hu WC, Chang YH. Evaluation of scalp and auricular acupuncture on EEG, HRV, and PRV. The American Journal of Chinese Medicine. 2007;**35**(02):219-230

[24] Yuan Q , Ma RL, Zhang JW, Jin R. Effect of acupuncture on cerebral images in autism children. World Journal of Acupuncture - Moxibustion. 2004;**14**(3):3-8

[25] Bao CL, Zhang LR, Dong GR. Effect of scalp penetration acupuncture on plasma level of ET-1 and NSE in patients with acute intracerebral hemorrhage. Journal of Clinical Acupuncture and Moxibustion. 2005;**21**:21-22

[26] Broyd SJ, Demanuele C, Debener S, Helps SK, James CJ, Sonuga-Barke EJ. Default-mode brain dysfunction in mental disorders: A systematic review. Neuroscience and Biobehavioral Reviews. 2009;**33**(3):279-296

[27] Si QM, Wu GC, Cao XD. Effects of electroacupuncture on acute cerebral infarction. Acupuncture & Electro-Therapeutics Research. 1998;**23**(2):117-124

[28] Yi G, Wang J, Bian H, Han C, Deng B, Wei X, et al. Multi-scale order recurrence quantification analysis of EEG signals evoked by manual acupuncture in healthy subjects. Cognitive Neurodynamics. 2013;**7**(1):79-88

[29] Dhond RP, Kettner N, Napadow V. Neuroimaging acupuncture effects in the human brain. The Journal of Alternative and Complementary Medicine. 2007;**13**(6):603-616

[30] Samuels N, Gropp C, Singer SR, Oberbaum M. Acupuncture for psychiatric illness: A literature review. Behavioral Medicine. 2008;**34**(2):55-64

[31] Franco-Santana LE, Torres-Castillo S, González-Trujano ME, González-Ramírez M. Stimulation of the Po-shen and Shen-hun scalp-acupuncture bands modifies levels of inhibitory and excitatory amino acids in the immature rat brain. Neurochemistry International. 2013;**63**(4):275-282

[32] Zhang XJ, Wu Q. Effects of electroacupuncture at different acupoints on learning and memory ability and PSD-95 protein expression on hippocampus CA1 in rats with autism. Zhongguo zhen jiu= Chinese acupuncture & moxibustion. 2013;**33**(7):627-631

[33] Gao XY, Ma QL, Hu B. Effects of acupuncture at "Sishencong" (EX-HN 1) on physiological functions in the sleep disorder model mouse. Zhongguo zhen

jiu= Chinese acupuncture & moxibustion. 2007;**27**(9):681-683

[34] Weinberger AH, Gbedemah M, Martinez AM, Nash D, Galea S, Goodwin RD. Trends in depression prevalence in the USA from 2005 to 2015: Widening disparities in vulnerable groups. Psychological Medicine. 2018;**48**(8):1308-1315

[35] Horowitz S. Acupuncture for treating mental health disorders. Alternative and Complementary Therapies. 2009;**15**(3):135-141

[36] Luo H, Meng F, Jia Y, Zhao X. Clinical research on the therapeutic effect of the electro-acupuncture treatment in patients with depression. Psychiatry and Clinical Neurosciences. 1998;**52**(S6):S338-S340

[37] Smith CA, Armour M, Lee MS, Wang LQ , Hay PJ. Acupuncture for depression. The Cochrane database of systematic reviews. 4 Mar, 2018;**3**:CD004046

[38] Grant S, Colaiaco B, Motala A, Shanman R, Sorbero M, Hempel S. Acupuncture for the treatment of adults with posttraumatic stress disorder: A systematic review and meta-analysis. Journal of Trauma & Dissociation. 2018;**19**(1):39-58

[39] Van den Noort M, Yeo S, Lim S, Lee SH, Staudte H, Bosch P. Acupuncture as add-on treatment of the positive, negative, and cognitive symptoms of patients with schizophrenia: A systematic review. Medicine. 2018;**5**(2):29

Chapter 5

Ultrasound Detection Acupuncture Needling Training: Description of the Method

Ying-Ling Chen and Mark C. Hou

Abstract

Acupuncture is unique to Chinese medicine and is widely used in practice. In order to avoid the complication of pneumothorax due to needle puncture of the lungs, we developed an ultrasound detection acupuncture (UDA) approach to measure the safe needle depth to improve patient safety. This study established a UDA training program and recruited trainees in our hospital to validate the effectiveness of the program. The trainees attended an eight-hour course, and practiced their skills using an acupuncture simulator model of GB21. Pre- and post-test data were analyzed. The level of satisfaction of the trainees was assessed by interview. In total, 16 trainees completed the course. Kendall's coefficient for the program was 0.82, and the average CVI was 0.98, showing good reliability and validity. Trainees exhibited significant improvement in terms of reduction of the incidence of pneumothorax after completing the course (P < 0.05), and the trainees were satisfied with the teaching of the ultrasound skill. Feedback from interviews showed that use of ultrasound to measure the safe needle depth may improve the mastery of acupuncture point GB21 and reduce the fear of causing pneumothorax.

Keywords: acupuncture, ultrasound, medical education, patient safety

1. Introduction

Acupuncture is a technique that is unique to Traditional Chinese medicine for treating illness and improving health [1]. Since it was introduced to Western countries in the 1970s, acupuncture has been widely-studied using modern clinical research approaches. In 2000, a large-scale acupuncture clinical trial was conducted in Germany due to controversy over insurance reimbursements for acupuncture treatment. According to the results of the trial, acupuncture was found to be valuable for pain relief, benefiting patients with back pain, knee pain and headache. In 2002, the World Health Organization (WHO) conducted a review of the results of controlled clinical trials, and concluded that the indications for acupuncture can be classified into four groups of disorders. The first group is diseases, symptoms or conditions for which acupuncture has been proved to be an effective management technique through controlled trials. There are 28 disorders belonging to this group, including stroke, lower back pain, headache, and hypertension [2]. In recent years, more clinical trials have been performed in patients with other disorders, such as dysmenorrhea [3]. Although the scientific community does not yet completely understand the mechanism of acupuncture, its efficacy is widely-accepted worldwide.

As with most medical interventions, acupuncture can also cause varying degrees of side effects. In a study by White [4], the risk of adverse events occurring in association with acupuncture was found to be very low when performed by qualified practitioners. As some serious adverse events may cause life-threatening complications, it is very important to actively prevent serious side effects. Common acupuncture side effects include pain at the punctured region, ecchymosis or hematoma, lightheadedness/dizziness, and pneumothorax [4–7]. With the exception of lightheadedness/dizziness, which is more relevant to the patient's physiological condition during acupuncture, the adverse events are related to the practitioner's technique and the depths of needles at acupoints. Among the major acupuncture-related adverse events, pneumothorax is the most severe, and therefore it is crucial that acupuncture practitioners identify safe depths of insertion of acupuncture needles for individual patients. Studies by Professor Lin and colleagues have extensively investigated the safe needle depth [8–12]. In one study of 11 acupuncture points in the neck and shoulder region, they found that the mean depths for the points around the shoulder in all study subjects, regardless of BMI and gender, were as follows: GB21 = 5.6 cm, SI14 = 5.2 cm, and SI15 = 8.8 cm. Subjects with a higher BMI had greater measured depths for most points [9]. However, the researchers also pointed out that differences between individuals are present, and it is difficult to set a standard. Therefore, study has been performed using modern imaging techniques, such as tomography, nuclear magnetic resonance, and ultrasonography, to directly measure the safe needle depths at acupuncture points in patients [12]. Ultrasound-guided aspiration has been widely-used to remove extra fluid from parts of the body, such as paracentesis of ascitic fluid, thoracentesis of pleural fluid [13], insertion of small-bore chest tubes in patients on clopidogrel [14], and placement of a central venous catheter [15]. Ultrasound-aided procedures are non-invasive, and the device is easy to access and relatively simple to operate. It is therefore the most suitable technique for detecting the needle depth during acupuncture. When practitioners perform acupuncture at dangerous acupoints, ultrasound imaging can help to identify the safe needle depth and prevent damage to organs. We named this technique, which combines acupuncture with ultrasound, ultrasound detection acupuncture (UDA). Taking acupoint GB21 (Jianjing; Gallbladder 21) in the chest area as an example, ultrasound was first used to measure the distance from the skin surface at the acupoint to the pleura, and the safe needle depth at the acupoint was then defined as a distance shorter than the one measured. In this way, pneumothorax can be avoided by preventing the needle from puncturing the lung or pleural cavity, which improves the safety and quality of treatment.

This study aimed to integrate the ultrasound technique into acupuncture training, and developed a course that teaches the use of ultrasound to measure the safe needle depth at difficult acupoints (e.g., GB21). We created a model of an acupoint for the course participants to practice on, and evaluated the efficacy of the training by qualitative and quantitative assessment.

2. Educational efficacy of an ultrasound detection acupuncture program

2.1 Materials and methods

2.1.1 Participants

This study was approved by the Institutional Review Board of our hospital (IRB No.: 151211) before the study was initiated. Residents in our hospital were recruited,

| Recruitment and consent |
| Pre-test and interview |
| 4 ultrasound acupuncture classes, 8 hrs in total |
| Post-test and interview |

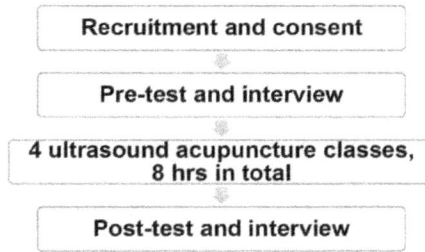

Figure 1.
Study flow chart.

the inclusion criterion being medical residents of the Department of Chinese Medicine who volunteered to participate in the training course. The participants were informed in detail about the training and completed a consent form before the start of the course. As the residents were trainees, which constitute a vulnerable group, and therefore in order to safeguard their rights, the recruitment process was publicly announced, and there was no mentor-trainee or colleague relationship between the recruiter and potential participants in order to ensure that the participants joined the study completely of their own accord.

After enrollment in the study, a pre-test and an interview were carried out for each participant, followed by a program of four 2-h ultrasound acupuncture training classes. After completion of the course, a post-test and another interview were performed to assess the efficacy of the training (**Figure 1**).

2.1.2 Development of the ultrasound detection acupuncture program

2.1.2.1 Design

A preliminary draft of the course was designed by ultrasound clinicians, clinical acupuncturists, and medical education experts, and then reviewed by a committee comprising five Chinese medical physicians qualified to teach in traditional Chinese medicine medical institutions under the regulations implemented by The Ministry of Health and Welfare, Taiwan. Course standards and DOPS (Direct Observation Procedural Skills) were then established to assess trainee skills.

Four experts were invited to serve as lecturers for the program. After the initial course content had been established, two lecturers generated teaching slides, and a test course was taught to two students. The students were then asked to provide feedback in order to improve the course, and the review committee also gave suggestions on the revision of the teaching content, enabling completion of the first draft of the course.

Next, we generated a questionnaire, which was reviewed by the five members of the review committee. The questionnaire was then revised until it passed validity and reliability testing, and the teaching content was modified to obtain the final teaching materials for the program. The classes of the program were taught by four lecturers (**Figure 2**).

Meeting agenda for course planning:

1. Clinical experience of dangerous acupoints.

2. Discussion of the ultrasound technique to be taught in the course.

3. Design of DOPS as the tool to assess the effectiveness of the course (**Table 1**).

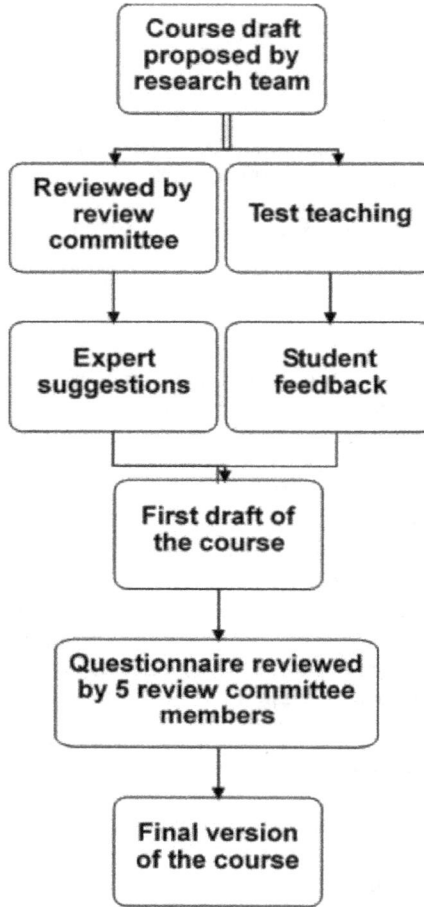

Figure 2.
Establishment of the ultrasound detection acupuncture course.

DOPS is an assessment tool developed by the Royal College of Physicians that is used to evaluate the performance of a trainee in learning a practical procedure in the United Kingdom [16]. This study used DOPS to assess the performance of the students after taking the course.

2.1.2.2 Ultrasound acupuncture course content

1. Principles and operation of ultrasound (2 h): this module of the course introduced the principles of ultrasonography in diagnosis, its use in visualizing different tissues and organs, and advanced medical ultrasound. The trainees learned the configuration and operation of a Sonosite ultrasound machine (model: NanoMaxx; Fujifilm Sonosite Inc), and had hands-on practice on an acupuncture simulator model of GB21 (ASM21), in addition to practice on a human body.

2. Patient safety and safe needle depth (2 h): clinical requirements and precautions for patient safety, introduction to simulation training, and the importance of improving patient safety.

Evaluation items	Under expected standard	Close to expected standard	Achieved expected standard	Over expected standard	Total
1. Ability in acupoint identification and acupoint selection.	☐ 1 ☐ 2	☐ 3	☐ 4	☐ 5 ☐ 6	☐
2. Ultrasound operation skills	☐ 1 ☐ 2	☐ 3	☐ 4	☐ 5 ☐ 6	☐
3. Suitable needle length selection before procedure	☐ 1 ☐ 2	☐ 3	☐ 4	☐ 5 ☐ 6	☐
4. Whether needle is placed in the correct acupoint area (simulator model sensor light on)	☐ 1 ☐		☐ 4		☐
5. Whether needle punctured the lung, causing pneumothorax (simulator model alarm light on)	☐ 1 ☐ 2		☐ 4		☐
6. Whether acupuncture procedure was completed within the set test time	☐ 1 ☐ 2	☐ 3	☐ 4	☐ 5 ☐ 6	☐
7. Overall assessment	☐ 1 ☐ 2	☐ 3	☐ 4	☐ 5 ☐ 6	☐
				Total score/ average	/

Table 1.
Scoring standard for acupuncture at GB21 using the direct observation of procedural skills (DOPS) tool.

3. Advanced clinical application for GB21 (2 h): the function and anatomical position of the acupoint GB21, its possible complications and their management.

4. Introduction and practice for ASM21 (2 h): the configuration of the ASM21 model and its function. The benefit and improvement in clinical skills when used in combination with ultrasonography. The importance of implantation of simulation in learning.

In this study, GB21 was used as the target acupoint, and ASM21, an acupuncture simulator model of GB21, was developed to help the trainees to easily manage this acupoint (**Figure 3**). The ASM21 model was designed with a sensor that detected whether the needle was placed in the correct position and within a safe depth, and an alarm sounded when the needle reached the lung. As it was constructed with material that is penetrable by ultrasound, the trainees could also measure the safe needle depth when the model was used together with an ultrasound machine.

2.1.2.3 Reliability of the ultrasound acupuncture course

We used the inter-rater reliability and employed Kendall's coefficient of concordance (W) for statistical analysis according to the scores given by the raters, as shown below:

$$W = \frac{R_i^2 - 1\frac{(R_i)^2}{N}}{\frac{1}{12}K^2(N^3 - N)} \qquad (1)$$

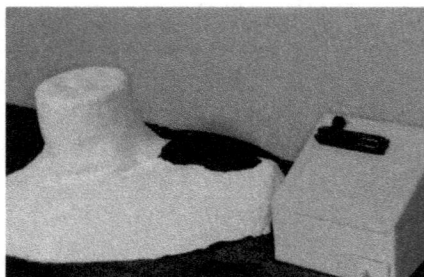

Figure 3.
Acupuncture simulator model of GB21 (ASM21) equipped with a sensor detector light alarm.

Where R_i^2 = the total sum of the squares of the scores given by the raters; $(R_i)^2$ = the square of the sum of the scores from each rater; N = number of trainees being evaluated; K = number of raters (experts).

We analyzed the W values of the trainees in the four classes. W values greater than 0.8 indicated good reliability.

2.1.2.4 Validity of the ultrasound acupuncture course

The course validity was calculated using the content validity index (CVI). The CVI method determines the ratio of experts who are in agreement with one another, and allows several raters to independently review the test items and evaluate the performance of the trainees. Briefly, for each test item, a scale of 4 was used for the rater response, responses of 1 and 2 indicating items that are 'invalid', and responses of 3 and 4 indicating 'valid' items. During the analysis, the four ordinal response rankings were then collapsed into two dichotomous categories of responses (score of invalid item = 0; score of valid item = 1), and the CVI of individual items was obtained. The CVI of the overall scale (S-CVI) was then calculated as:

$$S - CVI = \frac{CVI_i}{N} \tag{2}$$

where CVI_i is the sum of individual item CVIs and N is the total number of items. An S-CVI of 0.8 or higher indicated an acceptable validity. This study used IBM SPSS version 25 for quantitative statistical analysis.

2.1.3 Effectiveness assessment

2.1.3.1 Evaluation process

1. Pre-test: the trainees conducted acupuncture at the GB21 acupoint using the ASM21 model without ultrasound, and the frequency of occurrence of pneumothorax (needle puncture of the lung) was recorded on the DOPS form.

2. Pre-test interview: interviews were conducted with the trainees, which focused on acupuncture clinical skills and recorded their thoughts on and difficulties in performing acupuncture at the GB21 acupoint.

3. The trainees attended four classes, totaling an eight-hour course. They were asked to complete a satisfaction survey, and undertook two acupuncture practice sections with ultrasound.

4. Post-test: the trainees performed acupuncture at the GB21 acupoint using the ASM21 model without ultrasound, and the frequency of pneumothorax was recorded.

5. Post-test interview: interviews were conducted with the trainees to record their learning experience and thoughts.

6. Ultrasound acupuncture technical operation procedure: (i) identify GB21 on ASM21; (ii) use ultrasound to measure the distance from the surface to the lung, and use a depth shorter than this measurement as the safe needle depth; (iii) select a needle of appropriate length (the needle body must not exceed the above recorded depth); (iv) use a 28-gauge stainless steel acupuncture needle to perform the procedure; and (v) the test duration was defined from the first use of the needle to when the needle reached GB21 or punctured the lung.

2.1.3.2 Analyses of the results

The pre-test and post-test data were compared. Trainee feedback was also analyzed in order to evaluate the efficacy of the course using the methods described below:

1. Test methods: due to the small number of samples, and the fact that the data were not normally distributed, the Mann-Whitney U test and Fisher's exact test were used to determine whether the trainee skills at GB21 improved after taking the course.

2. Comparison of attendance and performance: the number of times that the needle punctured the lung was compared with the attendance rate by Fisher's exact test.

3. Effect of ultrasound class attendance: the number of times that the needle punctured the lung was compared with the attendance rate at the ultrasound class using Fisher's exact test.

4. Effect of ultrasound skills: the number of times that the needle punctured the lung was compared with the trainee's ultrasound skills using Fisher's exact test.

5. Practice and performance: the relationship between practice and performance was examined by comparing the trainees' practice simulations and the number of times that puncture of the lung occurred using Fisher's exact test.

6. Practice and ultrasound skills: whether the improvement in ultrasound skills was correlated with the number of practice sessions was examined using Fisher's exact test.

2.2 Results

2.2.1 Trainee recruitment

The study recruited 17 trainees, all of whom were residents at the Chinese Medicine Department of our hospital. One of the trainees was not able to attend all the classes and complete the test; therefore, a total of 16 participants, 8 males and 8 females (aged 31.63 ± 4.46 years), completed the program and were included in this study. Of them, one was a dual-licensed Chinese and Western medical physician, and the remaining 15 were all licensed Chinese medical practitioners (**Table 2**).

2.2.2 Ultrasound detection acupuncture course

2.2.2.1 Expert advice given during course planning meetings and feedback from trainees

During course planning, several experts suggested that more detailed information about the clinical effects of the advanced application of the GB21 acupoint should be introduced to the trainees, and a half-hour practice session for acupoint selection should be added to the course. As ultrasonography is a relatively unfamiliar technique for Chinese medicine practitioners, in addition to the principles taught in class, the experts also recommended that the trainees be given extra time to practice using the ultrasound machine as per the individual needs of the trainees. The identification of suitable teaching staff for the technique was also important and the process of selection of teaching staff needed to be confirmed.

2.2.3 Reliability and validity analyses

Reliability was determined according to the W value of the questionnaires from the raters. A W value of 0.821 was obtained, and the inter-rater reliability was between 0.71 and 0.9 ($P < 0.05$), suggesting that the five raters had a high degree of consistency in scoring the performance of the trainees. The results indicated that the ultrasound-guided acupuncture course had an excellent reliability and the design of the teaching materials was appropriate.

The S-CVI values of the five experts were 1, 1, 1, 0.9, and 1, all higher than 0.80, with an overall average of 0.98. This demonstrated that the course had an excellent validity, and that the course design achieved a high standard (**Table 3**).

Based on the results of the course planning meeting, as well as the reliability and validity analyses, the ultrasound-guided acupuncture course was designed to include four modules, which were taught in four different classes: "Introduction and operation of ASM21", "Advanced clinical application of the GB21 acupoint", "Patient safety and safe acupuncture needle depth", and "Principles and application of ultrasonography".

	n	Percentage (%)
Gender		
Male	8	50
Female	8	50
Age (years)		
21–30	7	43.75
31–40	8	50
>41	1	6.25
Had Western medical license	1	6.25

Table 2.
Demographic information of the trainees in this study

2.2.4 Assessment of student learning effectiveness

In the pre-test, the trainees had not learned the ultrasound technique, and therefore item 2—"Ultrasound operation skills" was not included for evaluation on the DOPS form. The average DOPS score in the pre-test was 3.0 ± 0.6. After the 16 trainees had attended the four classes, the average post-test score, which included item 2, was 3.8 ± 0.3. The Mann-Whitney U test (two-tailed) showed that the scores differed significantly between pre- and post-test ($P < 0.05$; **Table 4**). Overall, the use of ultrasound effectively helped the trainees to avoid the complication of pneumothorax when performing acupuncture at the GB21 acupoint.

2.2.5 Pre- and post-test interviews

The pre-test interviews indicated that most of the trainees did not have experience in performing acupuncture at the GB21 point prior to taking this course, and were afraid of causing pneumothorax when performing acupuncture at acupoints near to the chest. To assess the satisfaction of the trainees following the course, they were asked to complete a questionnaire after each class. For the four classes, 8, 10, 14, and 12 completed questionnaires were received.

Feedback was also obtained from the trainees during the post-test interviews, and some useful suggestions were collected as a reference to improve the program, as listed below (**Figure 4**).

2.2.6 Correlations between course attendance and post-test results

In this program, the trainees were free to participate in the classes according to their individual schedules. Due to the fact that the working hours and locations of the hospital residents might change, some trainees were unable to attend the entire course. The attendance rate and frequency of practice using the ultrasound instrument are presented in **Table 5**. When a trainee was not able to attend a class, video recordings and slides were provided for self-learning. Of the original 17 trainees recruited to this study, one withdrew; therefore, the data of 16 trainees were included for analysis.

Expert no.	S-CVI value
1	1
2	1
3	1
4	0.9
5	1
Average	0.98

Table 3.
S-CVI values obtained from the five experts as raters in this study.

	Pre-test (n = 16)	Post-test (n = 16)	P-value
Average score	3.0 ± 0.6	3.8 ± 0.3	0.00054[*]

Table 4.
Comparison of pre- and post-test scores by the Mann-Whitney U test (two-tailed).

Nine trainees attended the "Introduction and operation of ASM21" class (attendance rate = 56%); 12 trainees attended the "Advanced clinical application of GB21" class, but one left early (attendance rate = 69%); 12 participated in the "Patient safety and safe needle depth" class (attendance rate = 75%); and 15 participated in the "Principles and application of ultrasonography" class, but one left early (attendance rate = 88%). The average attendance rate was $75 \pm 0.25\%$. The total number of trainees who practiced using the ultrasound instrument was 12, accounting for 75% of the total number of participants (**Table 5**).

There was no incidence of puncture of the lung during use of the ASM21 model. To test whether attendance at the course was correlated with post-test performance, Fisher's exact test was performed, and showed that P = 1.0, indicating that class attendance had no significant association with the incidence of lung puncture. Additionally, analysis of the relationship between attendance at Class 4 ("Principles and application of ultrasonography") and the incidence of lung puncture also demonstrated that no correlation existed (P = 1.0). Further analysis indicated that acquisition of a good ultrasound technique reduced the incidence of lung puncture (P < 0.05), suggesting that acquisition of ultrasound skills helped to prevent

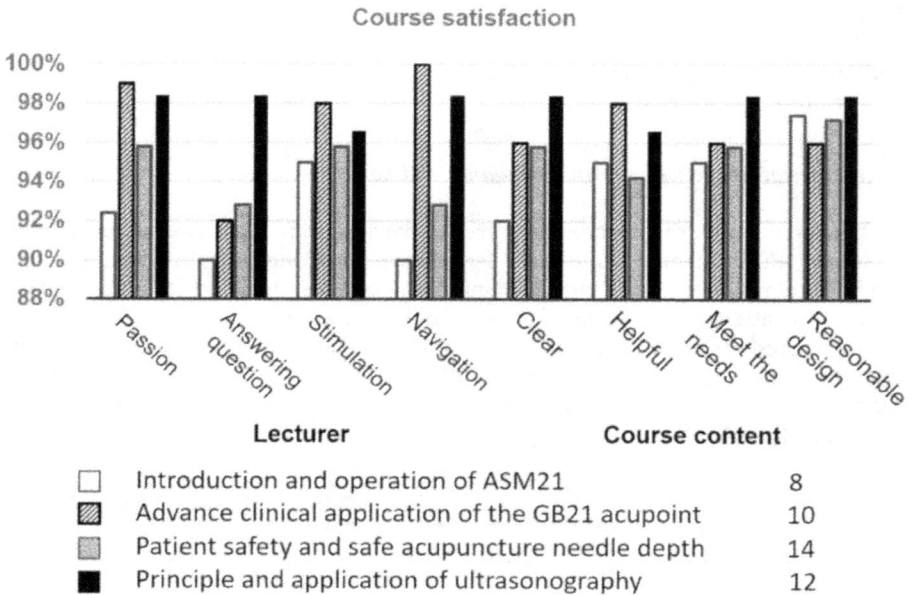

Figure 4.
Course satisfaction survey.

Item	P-value
Attending all classes *vs.* performance	1
Attending ultrasound class *vs.* lung puncture	1
Acquisition of ultrasound skills *vs.* lung puncture	1.6121e−05[***]
Practice using ultrasound instrument *vs.* lung puncture	1

Fisher's exact test ([***]*P < 0.001).*

Table 5.
Correlation analyses of trainee course attendance with post-test results.

pneumothorax post-test. Finally, no significant relationship was found between practice using the ultrasound machine and puncture of the lung.

Correlation between practice using the ultrasound instrument and improvement of ultrasound skills.

According to the second item (ultrasound skills) on the DOPS scale (score range = 1–6), the post-test score distribution of the trainees was 3–5. Three trainees had a score of 3 (2 had practiced using the instrument, 1 had not); 12 trainees had a score of 4 (9 had practiced, 3 had not), and one had a score of 5 (who had practiced). Fisher's exact test showed that practice using the ultrasound instrument was not correlated with improvement of ultrasound skills. In the post-test, the depth measurements at acupoint GB21 obtained by seven trainees were 3.0, 3.0, 3.2, 3.3, 3.5, 3.8 and 5.0 cm; the average depth was 3.5 ± 0.7 cm, which was very close to the actual depth of 3.5 cm. The depth measurement of 5.0 cm was much larger than the

Class	Case numbers	Interview key content
General	107010818010	I used to utilize oblique insertion and avoid dangerous acupuncture points. Now, I am glad that ultrasound can assist practitioners in precisely placing acupuncture needles, and reduce the fear of performing acupuncture at difficult points. In order to make this course more meaningful, I suggest having a qualifying examination after the course
Class 1: introduction and operation of ASM21	107010918005	Trainees were curious about using the ASM21 model to practice acupuncture ASM21 allows us the opportunity to practice very well at GB21. As GB21 is not often used clinically, performance in reality is rarely seen. I am looking forward to practicing at this point. Patient safety has always been an important principle in medical ethics
Class 2: advanced clinical application of the GB21 acupoint	107020618004	Trainees had the opportunity to further understand the timing of using GB21, and learn how pneumothorax can occur and its management Training helped us to understand that a needle at the acupuncture point GB21 will reach the pleura at a certain depth (about 2–3 cm), and insertion of the needle to a deeper position will penetrate the lung. Studies from Western medicine also showed that even anesthesia cannot block the pain at this point
Class 3: patient safety and safe acupuncture needle depth	107030818012	Trainees improved their knowledge of the safe needle depth, and learned about pneumothorax complications caused by acupuncture from cases of evidence-based medicine Learning of personal experience from the lecturer about acupuncture-caused pneumothorax was impressed. This highlighted that the needle depth is critical during acupoint selection in clinical practice
Class 4: principles and application of ultrasonography	107040918001 107040918012	Following hands-on operation, the trainees gave positive feedback on the use of ultrasound to detect the safe needle depth for acupuncture The ultrasound device is simple and easy to use, and effectively prevents pneumothorax. It was a novel experience to use ultrasound, especially its application in acupuncture in the clinical setting

Table 6.
Interview records from trainees.

other measurements, and the trainee who made this measurement had not practiced using the ultrasound instrument and had a poor ultrasound skills score. If this outlier value was removed, the average depth was 3.3 ± 0.3 cm.

The average duration of operation of the ultrasound instrument by the trainees was 87 ± 42 s (ranging from 45 s to 2 min and 9 s).

2.2.7 Post-test interview

After attending the course, the trainees expressed that it helped them to reduce their fear of performing acupuncture at the GB21 point, and practice using the ASM21 model helped to improve their self-confidence. Some positive feedback received is presented below:

With the assistance of ultrasound, the depth of the GB21 point can be easily identified. It helps to choose the correct length of needle. By using a proper needle, it prevents causing the problem of puncturing the lung (10704201801001) (**Table 6**).

During the pre-test, I did not know what I was doing as I was full of fear. I never perform acupuncture at the GB21 point, and was therefore very nervous. During the post-test, I felt it was quite an interesting task, as I am more self-confident and can perform it immediately without delay (10704201800901).

When I perform acupuncture at points in the chest, I will double-check by using ultrasound, especially if the patient is elderly, a young woman or a child (10704201801703).

I wish that ultrasound could be more popularized. I will use it in the clinic, especially at those acupuncture points with a high risk of causing an accident. For the common points, I will not use it as it takes time to use it (10704201800203).

2.3 Discussion

UDA is an innovative acupuncture technique. It employs modern ultrasound technology to inject new vitality into this ancient medical system. UDA may reduce the risk of complications at difficult acupoints, such as pneumothorax. It can improve patient safety, and render acupuncture at several important but difficult and less-used acupoints (e.g., Gaohuangshu BL-43, and Back-Shu points) more easily performed by acupuncture practitioners. This will help the advantages of traditional acupuncture to be restored and preserved.

In this study, we developed a program that employed ultrasound technology during training in the use of difficult acupuncture points. In the course described in this study, the focus was the Jianjing point GB21. The course included four 2-h classes: "Introduction and operation of ASM21", "Advanced clinical application of GB21", "Patient safety and safe needle depth", and "Principles and application of ultrasonography". The design of the course aimed not just to teach trainees to operate the ultrasound instrument and the ASM21 model, but also to educate them about patient safety and the safe needle depth at the GB21 acupoint.

According to the satisfaction survey completed by the trainees who undertook the course, the trainees showed high interest in two of the classes in particular: "Advanced clinical application of GB21" and "Principles and application of ultrasonography". This might be due to these two classes being directly correlated with clinical application, while the other two classes were related to simulation education and medical quality, which hospital residents are often less interested in. In the post-test interviews, most of the trainees were positive about integrating the ultrasound technique into the teaching of acupuncture. As ultrasound imaging helps them to clearly identify the position of the lungs, it improved their confidence in performing acupuncture at the GB21 point. Most of the trainees who attended the course expressed that if the hospital could provide an ultrasound instrument at their out-patient clinic, they would be willing to apply the UDA knowledge they had learned from the course in patient practice.

Currently, the largest barrier to Chinese medicine practitioners or acupuncturists using ultrasound is the high cost of the instrument. Even an entry-level new machine will cost more than $10,000 USD. At this moment, with the exception of large hospitals or medical centers, most small clinics are not able to afford to install this instrument at their practice locations. To solve this problem and enable UDA to be widely-used, the purchase of used ultrasound instruments is an option. Alternatively, the development of a low-cost, small-sized simple ultrasound instrument without an imaging function (such as the Butterfly IQ [17], which can easily detect the needle depth), should be considered.

Education in traditional Chinese medicine is still relatively conservative in comparison with modern medical education. Although acupuncture is considered a less invasive therapy, it does require thousands of hours of training to gain the proper skills. However, education in acupuncture still very rarely uses modern teaching aids to assist learning, and especially rarely uses simulation-based learning. These issues are in urgent need of improvement. This study utilized an innovative method that integrated a simulator that mimicked the chest body part and modern ultrasound technology to help trainees to learn how to safely perform acupuncture at the GB21 point. The UDA approach allows greater application of the traditional acupuncture points in therapy, as many of the difficult points are known to be very important, but it is difficult to master the necessary skills. We used UDA in acupuncture education, emphasizing patient safety, which differed from traditional acupuncture education, which mainly focuses on classroom teaching and observational learning [18, 19]. The outcomes of this study indicated that new teaching methods are required for education in acupuncture, as the conventional education system for acupuncture is known to have many problems and needs to be improved [20, 21].

The introduction of a body part model in acupuncture education is very useful for the learner. Body parts or organ sets have been created, and others have developed a 3-D interactive virtual environment, phantoms or integrated platforms to assist learners in acupuncture training [22–25]. However, such types of models or virtual training simulation systems still cannot provide sensations similar to those felt when practicing on the human body. We developed the ASM21 model using material that could be punctured by stainless steel acupuncture needles and that was penetrable by ultrasound. Integrating this material with a sensor detector and a light alarm, the goal was to allow the learners to practice on an object similar to a patient in clinic, and to measure the needle depth by ultrasound. Using a high-quality simulator with a realistic chest model, learners are able to perform sufficient practice before applying UDA in actual patients. Rehabilitation medicine has attempted to incorporate acupuncture as one of its therapy techniques, and has integrated acupuncture with the ultrasound technique [26]. However, that application mainly focuses on soft tissue-related diseases, such as muscle and tendon disorders. Neither patient safety nor the theory of the Meridians has been paid attention to. From a different aspect, in the present study, we used the theory of traditional Chinese medicine and considered patient safety to promote acupuncture modernization.

Although Chinese medicine has a long history, its modernization has followed a difficult path. In the development of the UDA training course, we had a great appreciation of the obstacles faced. Modern medicine is closely integrated with modern science; modern medicine keeps pace with the development of science-based technology, and new technology is used to develop new products and treatments to improve patient care. However, the majority of Chinese medicine practitioners do not pay attention to new technology. Many researchers have continued to work hard to improve this dilemma [27–29], while more Chinese medicine peers are still needed to join in the modernization. The ASM21 model developed in this study can be further improved to incorporate ultrasound techniques by collaborating with medical engineering manufacturers, which might create a new path for the development of technology for use in the application of Chinese medicine.

The outcomes of our study show promise. However, there were some limitations. First, this study was an educational study conducted in a single group, i.e., hospital residents, and was not a randomized controlled trial. The small sample size was also a limitation.

However, by using qualitative and quantitative analyses to validate the efficacy, the results are still valuable, and can be taken as a useful reference for developing similar courses. The significant improvement in score after the trainees had attended the course indicated a well-designed course, which can help to reduce the risk of pneumothorax, a complication of acupuncture at difficult chest acupoints. Both the attendance rate and practice of the ultrasound technique were independent of the reduction in the incidence of pneumothorax, suggesting that the use of ultrasound is key to reducing the incidence of this complication. As the operation of the ultrasound instrument is simple, no special repeat practice is required, which is a significant advantage of UDA that should be promoted in the future. The trainees only need to learn to measure the safe depth of the needle, rather than being familiar with diagnostic sonography. Based on the outcomes and the feedback obtained from the trainees, the course could be shortened by focusing on the operation of the ultrasound instrument and practice using the simulator. In terms of satisfaction, the post-test interviews demonstrated that the trainees gave the highest ratings for the course, indicating that the course design was successful.

In conclusion, a course design for acupuncture training needs to include practice using a simulator, which can greatly enhance the interest and motivation of the trainees. In the interviews, several trainees suggested that acupuncture clinical instructors should receive UDA training, which showed that they were not satisfied with the conventional educational approach. Some trainees also had different opinions to those of the lecturers for the classes, suggesting that the new generation no longer fully accepts the arrangements of traditional education. In order to achieve the goal of a high level of education, it is necessary to implement more communication between teachers and students in the current medical education setting.

3. Conclusion

3.1 UDA

UDA, by introducing ultrasound into acupuncture practice, will be a revolution technique for traditional acupuncture. UDA can not only reduce the risk of severe advertise effect when needing dangerous points, but also increase the usage of some important points traditionally, such as GB21 and BL43. We proposed the standard operating procedure for UDA and developed a course for UDA training. A video demonstration could be found at the web www.Dr-Hou.com. We truly hope that UDA would be widely accepted and performed popularly everywhere in acupuncture practice.

3.2 Future work

In order to prompt UDA further, a specific and affordable ultrasound devise is urgent needed. All the ultrasound devises available are too complicated and expensive for acupuncturists. We are currently in cooperation with medical engineers to develop a UDA special ultrasound. This ultrasound devise for safety depth (USD) will be a handy and useful devise specially designed to measure the safe needling distance of dangerous points. We believe that only by introducing and developing new ideas and practices can renew and update acupuncture. Thus an energetic and a fresh acupuncture can be presented to the world.

Acknowledgements

We like to thank Dr. Su-ChingLin, Dr. Jian-GuoBau, Dr. Bo-Shiu Chen, Dr.Yuen-Chun Lo, and Dr. Mao Sheng Sun for their help and inspirations. We also want to thank Miss Davy Kuo, Ariel Yu, and Sherry Ho. This study was funded by Ministry of Technology (no: MOST 106-2511-S-371-001) and Changhua Christian Hospital (no: 106-CCH-MST-133).

Conflict of interest

There is no financial relationship to disclose.

Author details

Ying-Ling Chen[1] and Mark C. Hou[2*]

1 China Medical University, Taichung, Taiwan

2 Changhua Christian Hospital, Changhua, Taiwan

*Address all correspondence to: dr.markhou@gmail.com

IntechOpen

References

[1] Hsu ES, Wu I, Lai B. Acupuncture. In: Essentials of Pain Medicine. Fourth Edition. 2018:545-550

[2] Organization WH. Acupuncture: Review and Analysis of Reports on Controlled Clinical Trials. Geneva: World Health Organization Available at: http://wwwiamaedu/OtherArticles/acupuncture_WHO_full_reportpdf; 2002 [Accessed Jan, 1 2018. 2016;31]

[3] Witt CM, Reinhold T, Brinkhaus B, Roll S, Jena S, Willich SN. Acupuncture in patients with dysmenorrhea: A randomized study on clinical effectiveness and cost-effectiveness in usual care. American Journal of Obstetrics and Gynecology. 2008; **198**(2):166. e1-166. e8

[4] White A. A cumulative review of the range and incidence of significant adverse events associated with acupuncture. Acupuncture in Medicine. 2004;**22**(3):122-133

[5] Melchart D, Weidenhammer W, Streng A, Reitmayr S, Hoppe A, Ernst E, et al. Prospective investigation of adverse effects of acupuncture in 97 733 patients. Archives of Internal Medicine. 2004;**164**(1):104-105

[6] Ernst G, Strzyz H, Hagmeister H. Incidence of adverse effects during acupuncture therapy—A multicentre survey. Complementary Therapies in Medicine. 2003;**11**(2):93-97

[7] Shinbara H, Ogasawara C, Hayama S, Hino K, Taniguchi H, Sumiya E. A survey of adverse events at acupuncture and moxibustion clinics in Japan. Journal of the American Medical Association. 2012;**2**:31-40

[8] Chou P-C, Huang Y-C, Hsueh C-J, Lin J-G, Chu H-Y. Retrospective study using MRI to measure depths of

acupuncture points in neck and shoulder region. BMJ Open. 2015;**5**(7): e007819

[9] Lin J-G, Chou P-C, Chu H-Y. An exploration of the needling depth in acupuncture: The safe needling depth and the needling depth of clinical efficacy. Evidence-Based Complementary and Alternative Medicine. 2013:1-21

[10] Chou P-C, Chu H-Y, Lin J-G. Safe needling depth of acupuncture points. The Journal of Alternative and Complementary Medicine. 2011;**17**(3): 199-206

[11] Chen H-N, Lin J-G, Ying L-C, Huang C-C, Lin C-H. The therapeutic depth of abdominal acupuncture points approaches the safe depth in overweight and in older children. The Journal of Alternative and Complementary Medicine. 2009;**15**(9):1033-1037

[12] Chen H-N, Lin J-G, Yang AD, Chang S-K. Safe depth of abdominal acupoints in pediatric patients. Complementary Therapies in Medicine. 2008;**16**(6):331-335

[13] Dattola A, Alberti A, Giannetto G, Di DM, Basile G. Echo-guided percutaneous drainage of abscesses and abdominal fluid collections. Annali Italiani di Chirurgia. 1999;**70**(2):161-167

[14] Dammert P, Pratter M, Boujaoude Z. Safety of ultrasound-guided small-bore chest tube insertion in patients on clopidogrel. Journal of Bronchology & Interventional Pulmonology. 2013; **20**(1):16-20

[15] Ajayi G. Ultrasonography-guided amniocentesis in singleton pregnancies: A review of the first 1,000 cases. Clinical and Experimental Obstetrics & Gynecology. 2011;**38**(4):405

[16] Wilkinson JR, Crossley JG, Wragg A, Mills P, Cowan G, Wade W. Implementing workplace-based assessment across the medical specialties in the United Kingdom. Medical Education. 2008;**42**(4):364-373

[17] ButterflyIQ. Meet IQ. Available from: https://www.butterflynetwork.com/

[18] Yeh GY, Ryan MA, Phillips RS, Audette JF. Doctor training and practice of acupuncture: Results of a survey. Journal of Evaluation in Clinical Practice. 2008;**14**(3):439-445

[19] Janz S, Adams J. Acupuncture education standards in Australia: A critical review. Australian Journal of Acupuncture and Chinese Medicine. 2011;**6**(1):3

[20] Flaws B. American acupuncture education: Has a wrong turn been taken? American Journal of Acupuncture. 1991;**19**(1):63-71

[21] Ijaz N, Boon H, Muzzin L, Welsh S. State risk discourse and the regulatory preservation of traditional medicine knowledge: The case of acupuncture in Ontario, Canada. Social Science & Medicine. 2016;**170**:97-105

[22] Heng P-A, Wong T-T, Yang R, Chui Y-P, Xie Y-M, Leung K-S, et al. Intelligent inferencing and haptic simulation for Chinese acupuncture learning and training. IEEE Transactions on Information Technology in Biomedicine. 2006;**10**(1):28-41

[23] Leung K-M, Heng P-A, Sun H, Wong T-T. A haptic needle manipulation simulator for Chinese acupuncture. Studies in Health Technology and Informatics. 2003: 187-189

[24] Lee I-S, Lee T, Shin W-C, Wallraven C, Lee H, Park H-J, et al.

Haptic simulation for acupuncture needle manipulation. The Journal of Alternative and Complementary Medicine. 2014;**20**(8):654-660

[25] Si W, Yuan Z-Y, Mao R, Zhao J, Liao X, Duan Z. Modeling and realization of virtual acupuncture training simulation system. JDCTA. 2010;**4**(8):126-136

[26] Litscher G. Modernization of traditional acupuncture using multimodal computer-based high-tech methods—Recent results of blue laser and teleacupuncture from the medical University of Graz. Journal of Acupuncture and Meridian Studies. 2009;**2**(3):202-209

[27] Litscher G, Huang T, Wang L, Zhang W. Violet laser acupuncture—Part 1: Effects on brain circulation. Journal of Acupuncture and Meridian Studies. 2010;**3**(4):255-259

[28] Wu J, Hu Y, Zhu Y, Yin P, Litscher G, Xu S. Systematic review of adverse effects: A further step towards modernization of acupuncture in China. Evidence-Based Complementary and Alternative Medicine. 2015:1-19

[29] Castro JA. Integrating acupuncture in the physical medicine and rehabilitation setting. Critical Reviews™ in Physical and Rehabilitation Medicine. 2005;**17**(4):301-316